# A
# STROKE
# *of* GRACE

*A Guide to Understanding and Living
With an Acquired Brain Injury*

*by*

## JULIANNE HEAGY

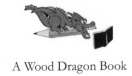

A Wood Dragon Book

**A Stroke of Grace**
– A Guide to Understanding and Living with
An Acquired Brain Injury

Cover design: Callum Jagger
Author photos by: Montana Falasca (MontanasPhotoWorks.com)
Interior design: Christine Lee

**Published by:**
Wood Dragon Books
Post Office Box 429
Mossbank, Saskatchewan, Canada S0H3G0
www.wooddragonbooks.com

Available in hardcover, paperback,
eBook and audiobook

ISBN: 978-1-989078-91-4 Hardcover
ISBN: 978-1-989078-89-1 Paperback
ISBN: 978-1-989078-90-7 eBook

**Author contact information**
Email: AStrokeOfGrace@sasktel.net
Mail: Post Office Box 880, Assiniboia, Saskatchewan,
Canada S0H0B0

# Dedication

*To my husband, Blair, who has been my caregiver, my friend, my confidant, my cheerleader, my rock and the greatest love of my life. Your calm, patience and understanding have made this journey more manageable.*

*To my dad, Alex Peter, who passed away April 28, 2021. He didn't have the opportunity to see my manuscript turn into a book. I trust he is watching over me and is proud of the work I have done.*

*To my children, Jared and Justine. Thank you for staying close and for always being loving and supportive—both with this book and life in general. I am so blessed.*

# *Table of Contents*

# PART FOUR

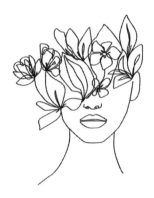

# Introduction

*"You don't think about your brain
until it's all you think about."*

I experienced a stroke on May 21, 2019.

Following my stroke, I felt very unsupported by the systems that should be in place to care for post-stroke victims. I knew there were resources available but with an inability to hold a thought or comprehend written words, I became angry and frustrated with my search for information. Aside from my family doctor, I seemed to be alone. Where were the people that would educate me so this wouldn't happen again? Where were the people that would tell me about therapies and services available to me? I knew some of these answers before my stroke but I couldn't recall the information I needed with my recently damaged brain.

As I began to heal, I could recall some of what I needed to know and committed to taking notes and sharing my findings with others on this same path. This book and its companion journal provide a roadmap of "What I have learned" on this journey.

The book is simply structured. The first section of the book is my first year's journal notes, and the next section is my second year's journal notes by calendar quarter. The third section of the book includes "Stepping Into Year Three" followed by "Things to Know About Someone with a Brain Injury … And How You Can Help" and "What Someone with a Brain Injury Would Tell Others if They Could."

Each chapter in the first segment includes "What I have learned," which provides links to resources, helpful hints on how to make your new life more manageable, and information on therapies and self-help strategies.

It goes without saying that no two people have the same experience with their stroke, subsequent brain injury and residual limitations. Everyone's recovery will be at their own pace and with varied results.

It is my firm belief that everything in our life happens for us and not to us. I wrote this book now because I've found improvement in my health, peace, and joy. I have always wanted to use my experience to help others. I knew that if my recovery would be sufficient to write this book (even though I'm not yet able to read it), my story could be the guiding roadmap that I so desperately wanted and needed in those early days after my stroke.

This book provides the information, easily and simply, for those struggling to ask the questions and find the resources. My goal is to educate, empower and encourage others with an acquired brain injury.

# PART ONE

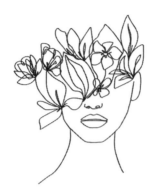

## Month 1
### (May 21–June 20, 2019)

It's Tuesday, May 21, 2019. As I awaken, I remember that this is the Tuesday following the Victoria Day long weekend and my desk at work awaits me with an abundance of things I need to do. I also remember that this is our 31st wedding anniversary, as well as the day of our daughter, Justine's, pharmacy licensing exam. *Lord, thank you for putting Blair in my life. Thank you for thirty-one years of ups and downs and especially for our ability to take every challenge and every victory to You in prayer. I especially pray for Justine this morning and ask that You give her peace. Lord, please bring the answers to the exam questions easily to her mind. I also ask that you keep Jared safe at work today. In Jesus' name I pray. Amen.* As my prayer ends, I recognize the roar of a car—

it belongs to our son, Jared; I can hear it every morning as he passes by our home on his way to work. I say a silent good morning to him and wish him a good day.

I move quietly around the condo as I get up and get dressed. My husband, Blair, was diagnosed with lung cancer six years ago and sleeps until 9:30 most mornings. He is stage IV but is doing remarkably well and has an amazingly positive attitude. Three times in the past six years we've been told he had less than ten months to live and each time he has "proven them wrong." His courage throughout this extremely difficult challenge inspires me. But the highs and lows of his cancer journey have been an emotional challenge for me and I'm so glad we're riding a high wave now. He has a PET scan every three months, and the most recent results showed a small concern. I try not to let it be a big worry.

I leave for work a little early to get a solid start on my day.

It's been a productive morning. I work as a Member Relations Officer at our local Co-op's head office in Assiniboia, Saskatchewan. The Co-op offers groceries, agricultural supplies, hardware, and fuel services. At this time of year, our administrative office is generally winding down following several major events, but we are still busy with presenting scholarships, handling requests for donations for summer events, and negotiating advertising with our new local radio station. My work schedule is always busy, but I thrive on keeping several balls in the air at once. I have much to do today, so I decide to eat lunch at my desk so that I can leave at five for our anniversary supper. I grab a salad from the deli in the grocery store downstairs.

I wonder how Justine's exam has gone and send up another quick prayer.

Text from Justine: *It's done. That's all I can say. Gonna go nap.*

At about 2:30, Blair texts and asks me to take a break for coffee with him at the local bakery just across the street from my office. Despite my workload, I decide to take a break. It's our anniversary and spending a few minutes together over a coffee is the least I can do. When I walk in, I'm surprised and thrilled to see Justine there. She had finished her exam before noon and had immediately started the three-hour drive from Saskatoon to surprise us for our anniversary

After this nice surprise, I head back to the office and try to prioritize what's still on my desk to see what I can accomplish before I head out for our supper. At coffee, we revised the plan from 'meeting at five' to 'leaving at 5:30.' I do some work, but I'm getting a bit of a headache. I have eaten only half of my salad. It really has been a long day. My eyes are starting to bother me. Little gold squares of light are in my field of vision.

5:19 p.m. — I am just not feeling great. I text Justine to ask her to bring her dad to the Co-op so he can drive my car home. I write: *Can you come to get me around with dad on 5:30. I'm very to delay.*
She replies: *You're delayed? You have the vehicle, remember? But I can* still come get you
I respond: *I don't think I can ride. Dad can take car home*
Justine: *OK. Are you OK?*
Me: *Not sure*

I know that Blair and Justine will be heading my way soon, so I decide to quickly contact some non-profit groups with the donations I've approved for them. The first request was for a donation of gift cards, but I can't think of the words "gift cards" to write on the donation request form. *It's been a long day,* I think. I'll come back to this request later. The next request was for a donation of beef. I decide it would be easier to just call the group, so I dial. Someone answers. I say, "Hi, this is…" and then I can't think of the next word. I feel like I'm in a big, dark, empty room and I can't find anything—not a word, not a thought, not an idea, just total blankness. I hear the person on the other end say, "from the Co-op?"

"Umhum." I'm so embarrassed by my response. What a

terrible representation of our Co-op.

"About our donation request?" the voice says.

"Umhum."

"Are you able to donate the beef?"

"Umhum."

"Thanks!"

I am so embarrassed during the call—wanting to hang up but thinking that would be even more rude than responding with a mumble. I want to cry! I look up and Blair is just entering the administration area on his way to my office. I'm feeling like my balance is off and I am realizing that it will be hard to walk down the stairs to the main floor and out to the parking lot.

The women at the administration desks wish us a happy anniversary and tell us to enjoy our evening. I smile and nod, and even offer a small wave as we leave. But I note Blair's forced smile and worried look.

I know I need Blair's support to get me down the stairs. Justine is waiting in the car and they take me to the local hospital. If I could speak, I would ask them to just take me home to sleep. I still think that I just don't feel well and am tired. Later, I find out that Blair and Justine knew I needed to go directly to Emergency.

I'm so glad to be able to lie down on the ER bed. I can

sense busyness around me, and I feel IVs going into both my arms. Having worked at this hospital periodically for over twenty years as a health information manager, an admitting and discharge clerk, and a casual scheduler, I know most of the nursing staff. I see concern in their eyes. They ask me my name but I can't find it in my mind; I get a quick glimpse of it, but then it's gone. When I do grasp it, I can't make my mouth work. I can't speak my name. I concentrate with all the effort I can muster and then it explodes out of me—my name, "Julianne." That was exhausting! Now I just want to rest. I have no thoughts in my head, no questions, and I feel no fear—I just have a desire to rest in the quiet emptiness.

Our family doctor has arrived and there is more commotion. They keep asking me my name. I hear someone say, "Blood pressure is 215 over 90."

I am being moved. The ambulance arrives to take me to the hospital in Moose Jaw—but I feel like I just arrived at this one. (Justine informs me later that the doctor said sometimes a migraine will take speech away temporarily but the treatment for the migraine would cause further vascular restriction so they didn't feel safe in treating me for migraine without a CT scan. So the decision was made to send me by ambulance to Moose Jaw.)

In the ambulance, I realize that I know my EMT. He

is the son of friends who were our best man and our organist at our wedding. They married the year after they met at our wedding. It feels good to see his kind, familiar face. (On reflection, I think that this is such a wonderful God-incident. Exactly thirty-one years ago, his parents met at our wedding. They dated, married, and created this compassionate, wise, and skillful young man who is now taking care of me.) He closely monitors my condition until I'm turned over to the hands of the physician at the next hospital.

The usual sixty-minute drive to Moose Jaw takes only forty minutes. Blair is with me in the ambulance, and Justine will meet us at the hospital.

At the Moose Jaw hospital, I sense another swirl of activity. Blood is being drawn and I'm being rushed for a CT scan. Shortly afterward, we receive the diagnosis of stroke. I don't feel fear, oddly; I just feel safe. The scan indicates it's not a brain hemorrhage, so I'm cleared to receive the tPA—the clot-buster—treatment. The scan also shows that I have a greater than 70 percent occlusion (or narrowing) of my left carotid artery. (Justine tells me later that I nod consent for the tPA treatment.) She has her pharmacy textbooks with her, and is busy researching stroke protocols. She gets in touch with Jared to tell him what is happening; he is over two hours away, but will come if I get any worse.

I must be in and out of sleep, or awareness, because all I remember is the nurses telling Blair and Justine that I'm to stay in bed for forty-eight hours as I am now a high bleed risk, from the tPA. Justine learns from the medical staff that the bleed risk is so high with this drug that I could bleed from my eyes.

I'm surprised to see the people around me in full protective gear and to find that I'm in an isolation room. My medical record history has shown that I was positive for ESBL (extended spectrum beta-lactamase), which is explained to us as being a superbug, possibly stemming from a previous bladder infection. I tested positive again on this admission and so I am in an isolation bed on the ICU ward. Thankfully Blair and Justine can be with me for comfort and to get information from the medical team.

The attending physician explains to us that I have been referred to a surgeon at the Regina General Hospital for a left carotid endarterectomy. The surgery entails opening my neck, opening the left carotid artery, scraping out the plaque, and then placing a patch on the carotid before closing me up. The surgery is to take place as soon as an isolation bed at Regina General is available. I must also stay in bed until the bleeding risk from the tPA treatment is over.

## *May 22*

At about 12:30 a.m., I waved and nodded to Blair and Justine that they should go home to rest. I am still unable to speak. Blair went home to Assiniboia and Justine to Limerick. (Justine later tells me that I showed great concern for Blair and his ability to stay awake and strong at this late hour.)

At 2 a.m., I'm feeling very chilled and want to ask for a blanket. I work hard to find the words to use when the nurse comes in to answer my buzzer. With all the effort I can muster, I blurt out, "Need a blanket." I start to cry, as does the nurse. My speech is back! What a huge relief. But I'm exhausted from working so hard to speak. The warm blanket is exactly what I need, and I fall back to sleep.

It's morning rounds. The ER doctor is very happy to hear that I have spoken during the night. Although it has become easier for me to find words, speaking is mentally tasking. I try hard though, because I want to know what happened to me. I ask the doctor if the stroke may have been caused by my low-carb, keto way of eating, as I had no other risk factors—I'm not a smoker, not diabetic, I don't have high cholesterol nor high blood pressure. He said, "Definitely not."

The dietitian is in to check on my ability to swallow before she can approve food. I am relieved when she requests a keto-friendly diet. Lunch is an egg salad sandwich wrapped in lettuce. I'm so grateful. More than anything, I feel that a low-carb diet helps to keep my anxiety in check. I began to experience anxiety as a frequent emotion after the death of my sister to cancer in 2009 and I didn't want to jeopardize my mental health.

We are still waiting for an isolation bed in Regina for the endarterectomy and I am still required to stay in bed until the bleeding risk from the tPA treatment is over. I am not even allowed to brush my teeth because of the bleeding risk. I'm also struggling with peeing into what looks like a cardboard bedpan. I have visions of it collapsing once it's wet. The struggle is real!

## *May 23 - May 24*

I slept and visited with family. Reading and watching TV is uncomfortable and is giving me headaches. I am feeling anxious regarding my lack of comprehension.

I am comforted to see that Blair plans to spend the night on a foldaway bed in my room.

In the next days, I am happy to see Jared, who comes to visit me and keeps in touch by phone. Justine is such a help. I am so grateful for their love and support.

I can walk, but I am unsteady. My vision is poor. I feel so tired.

## *May 25*

A bed is available at Regina General. Since I'm in pretty good physical shape at this point, the doctors have approved Blair to drive me as long as we go directly to the hospital.

I still feel off balance and sleep most of the trip.

As I settle into the new room, I am aware of how uncomfortable the IVs have become. I ask for extra pillows to prop my arms in a comfortable position. I am told there are no extra pillows. Eventually a nurse brings me a blanket I roll up and use to support my arm. That helps. The slip sheet under me has an old blood stain on it. I know it must have been washed, as the stain is faded, but I don't feel safe. I'm less than confident that I'm being well cared for. These thoughts are starting to consume me—maybe because my care in Moose Jaw had been exceptional. There is no attempt to accommodate a low-carb meal option here. In fact, the nurses laugh at my request and say that the majority of the meals are on the high-carb side.

We meet the surgeon. He explains that, without the surgery, a second stroke is imminent within the next few weeks—hence the request to go directly from the Moose Jaw hospital to one in Regina. My surgery is booked for May 27. He reviews the process of the endarterectomy exactly as it was explained to me earlier—open the left side of the neck, scrape out the plaque, apply a patch, and close the wound.

He asks, as did the other doctors, "Do you have diabetes? High blood pressure? High cholesterol? Are you a smoker?" I reply "No" to all these questions. He's curious to know—as we all are—why I have such a blockage when I have no risk factors. It is a question that may never be answered. Again, I ask if my keto way of eating may have contributed to the plaque build-up. He echoed the ER doctor and said, "Absolutely not." Again, I'm relieved to hear it. But I desperately want to know what I can do differently to avoid another blockage.

## *May 26*

I'm a little disturbed when the nurse comes in and asks me to swab myself for ESBL. She further instructs me to be sure to label the samples correctly. The swabs are to be taken from my nose, groin, and rectum. What? Why am I doing this? I'm not a nurse or lab tech. My vision and balance are not good. What about cross-contamination from swabbing all over the skin on my rear end until I'm able to find the "target"? This feels archaic to me, and my confidence in feeling safe here has dropped another notch.

## *May 27*

Today is my endarterectomy surgery. I still have the original IVs in both arms and they are very uncomfortable.

The intern comes in to brief me on the surgery. She explains that I will be in surgery for about half an hour and in recovery for approximately two hours. She further explains that another line will be inserted into my hand to monitor vessel pressure. Then, in the surgical suite, the intern attempts to insert the larger IV line, but she is struggling. The pain is almost unbearable. I begin to pray and silently sing to myself "The Garden," an old worship song I loved to play on the piano as a youth. The distraction is working. I am very relieved that the anesthetic is kicking in fairly quickly.

I fell asleep before the intern was able to successfully insert the IV, so I am not sure if she completed the task or if someone else did. I wake up after the surgery and immediately see that all the IVs have been restarted in new locations, and they feel more comfortable. I begin to check my body. My incision is about four inches long and goes from just under the upper corner of my left jaw and down my neck toward the front. There is also a drain in place at the top of my sternum/breast bone. I really have very little pain.

I'm very hungry but understand that my meal will be liquid until the dietitian confirms that I'm not a post-surgery choke risk. My supper arrives—perogies and sausage. I say that I was told to expect a liquid diet. The nurses say they'll see what they can find for me. In the meantime, Blair is enjoying my meal. No sense in it going to waste. The nurses never do come back with a liquid supper. I'm very slowly and carefully chewing the sausage because I'm so hungry.

My family is with me at various times throughout the day. Jared uses humour to cope with stress, and I appreciate it. Justine is a born caregiver and her medical training makes me feel safe as she discusses treatments and concerns with the physicians. Blair is my rock. Always calm and loving. I am so blessed.

Extreme headache tonight.

## *May 28*

The surgeon is in to check on me. He asks if I feel comfortable with going home after the drain is pulled today. *Yes!* I know I will feel safer at home.

He explains that the stroke was a brain injury, and that the surgery was a second assault to the brain. He suggests that I take my time with recovery. He says not to rush going back to work. I have already been worrying about all the work that needs my attention.

The trip home is quite comfortable. Soon I'm home and going to sleep, reclined on the couch with pillows propped on both sides of my head.

It feels so good to be in my home, to soak in my bath, and eat food that I want to eat. But I am very tired and feeling off-balance. I'm continuing to worry about work, and I call in to see if there is anything I can help with, just from my memory of which donation requests still need to be approved. My mental attention is short, but I'm able to help with a few questions.

I try to check my emails on the computer, but I'm experiencing visual disturbances. Sort of like looking through a kaleidoscope.

Constant dull headache.

## *May 31, 2019*

I am still experiencing fatigue, brain fog, and the feeling of being off-balance.

As a retired Registered Massage Therapist, a caregiver at heart, I feel desperate for help. I am expecting some aftercare that hasn't yet been offered. *Someone tell me what to do so this doesn't happen again! Someone tell me how to make my head stop hurting, my eyes to focus, my balance to come back so I can feel safe walking.*

During my short bursts of clarity, I get on the computer and search the Heart and Stroke Foundation of Canada website to see what I can find. It speaks of a handout that is given to every Canadian stroke victim before they leave the hospital. Nope! I didn't get one. I do see that I can print one.

Unfortunately, my reading comprehension is so poor that I'm able to get through only a page or two, but I appreciate that I will have some guidance when reading becomes easier.

I'm also grateful for my local community of massage therapists who have reached out with offers of treatments, including some therapies I have never heard of. Knowing from my massage training that massage is contraindicated (not to be used) for six weeks post-surgery, I decide to wait and just rest and heal for now.

Experiencing a lack of support and guidance is adding to my frustrations.

## *June 5 – June 7*

We are travelling to Saskatoon to attend Justine's convocation ceremony from the College of Pharmacy. To give me time for resting, we are going the day before the event. I have found a dress with a high collar to cover the scar and bruising on my neck. We are staying in a hotel very close to the graduation venue, allowing us to attend the ceremony in the morning and have lunch in our room, with food we brought.

Justine has always been goal-oriented. She has been a long-time student and has trained in kinesiology, massage therapy, pharmacy technology, and has now graduated as a pharmacist. I'm very proud to watch our beautiful daughter cross the stage and take on this new role.

After the ceremony, I sleep for the entire afternoon and feel quite rested for the banquet at five. I worry about my walking, and whether I chose the right shoes, but I hold tight to Blair as we walk. I even manage to stay awake until nine. At one point, I sit on a chair in the hallway to get away from the noise and visual stimulation; otherwise, I enjoy the evening. We are so very proud of our daughter's hard work. I wish Jared were able to get away from work to join us. We are glad to have Blair's parents, his sister, and our brother-in-law with us.

## *June 11*

Blair's telehealth meeting is this morning. We learn that he has a new tumour in his left lower lung lobe. The plan is to monitor it by PET scan, with the next one scheduled for September. The tumours found in his abdomen in March are unchanged. This emotional hit seems to tire my brain as much as any mental task does. I want him to be able to focus on his own health issues instead of now having to become my caregiver. *Please Lord, don't let this distraction and worry create a health crisis for him.*

I am still sleeping excessively and feel like my depth perception is off. Stairs are very hard to manoeuver. I feel like I'm in a fun house and the stairs and walls are moving and slanting. I can't read more than a couple of pages at a time, and my comprehension is poor; I am slow to process information.

## *June 20*

The power has been out all morning.

I am at my GP's for an appointment, and he is running an hour behind. I am very tired by the time I get in, and feel very chilled. I am so tired that I don't have the energy or the words to ask questions or express my concerns about the lack of aftercare. I do ask if the plaque in my neck would also be in my heart. The doctor tells me when I feel more stable on my feet, he will send me for a cardiac stress test.

Home to sleep. This outing has been exhausting.

As I look back on this first month after my stroke, I am at a loss to know what to do to get better. I know I should be moving my body, but I don't feel safe in doing so. I worry almost constantly and feel varying degrees of desperation.

Multi-tasking seems to overwhelm my brain—the physical indicators present as pressure, visual disturbances, and a general feeling of unwellness. Most of the time, my symptoms are relieved with sleep. Often, I hit the wall and experience extreme fatigue. Sleep comes quickly whenever I close my eyes.

I am not able to work, and we are feeling the consequential financial pinch. The good news is that being in stores makes me very dizzy, and if I am in a store too long I find it hard to find my words and to function—so at least that is a "budget-friendly" problem! I go into the office once a week for twenty to thirty minutes to help with the donation requests. I still felt a strong need and responsibility to help, and also want to avoid having a lot to catch up on when I return. I suppose this concern is a positive sign—to assume that I will be able to resume my work.

Numbers confuse me. For example, I planned to meet a friend for coffee at 10 a.m. When I looked at the clock at 9:19, I thought I had only 19 minutes to get ready and get to her house, which is 7 minutes away. I subsequently arrived quite early, and she was gracious in underplaying my mistake. I was at her door before I realized how my mind had twisted my timeline.

Overall, I feel desperate for help with how to move and manoeuvre in my newly limited world. *Please*, I would scream to myself, *What is happening with me? Someone tell me how to make this better!*

## *What I have learned ...*

Give yourself permission to rest. Your brain has been injured and needs time to heal. Be kind to yourself. The more you push to be on your computer, to read, to push past the fatigue, to carry on with your responsibilities at work, the more you are overstimulating the injured brain. As with any injured body part, there is inflammation. The purpose of inflammation is to tell your body that you're hurt and that you need to rest the injured part to help prevent re-injury.

I know this is hard—especially if you don't have any physical impairment after the stroke. I had a hard time convincing myself I was still "injured"—I couldn't see the damage, nor could friends and family. They assumed I was better because I could walk and talk. I so wanted them to be right.

**A stroke is serious business.** According to the Journal of Neuroinflammation, *"Stroke is a debilitating disease condition defined as either an interruption of blood supply to the brain due to a clot or embolism, or the rupture of a blood vessel in the brain, which then leads to neurological impairments. It remains the 3rd leading cause of death worldwide with nearly 15 million people being affected per year."* [1]

According to the Heart and Stroke Foundation of Canada, *"Stroke is on the rise. Ischemic stroke, caused by a blood clot, occurs in 85% of all stroke patients. A hemorrhagic stroke occurs in the remaining 15% when a blood vessel ruptures, causing bleeding in the brain. A transient ischemic attack (TIA) – sometimes referred to as a mini-stroke – is caused by a small clot that briefly blocks an artery. More than 62,000 strokes occur in Canada each year and that number continues to rise, leaving more than 405,000 people in Canada living with the effect of stroke."* (2)

**Being physically able to drive doesn't mean you should.** I found out well after the fact that if I had been driving and in a car accident in the first six months following my stroke, I would not have had any insurance coverage. Be sure to check your vehicle insurance for any restrictions you may have.

**Reach out to a physiotherapist.** Physiotherapists are direct-access practitioners, meaning patients can visit physiotherapists directly (using self-referral) without waiting for a physician referral. (3)

If you haven't already been referred, do yourself a favour and have a physio assessment. You may be unaware of residual weaknesses or imbalances. Now is the time to start your rehabilitation.

When you are approved for physical therapy, don't delay. Retraining the brain and muscles soon after a stroke is very important.

**Self-care is vital.** Rest, rest, rest. If your anxiety is worse now than it was in the past, it's okay to ask for help and speak with a counsellor. Learn what works for you; for example, for me, avoiding sugar helps to keep my anxiety down. Know that you have new limitations, as with any injury. Take time to rest and repair.

**Avoid self-medicating with drugs and alcohol.** Alcohol could interfere with any medicine you take to reduce your risk of having another stroke. In particular, alcohol can be harmful if you are taking blood-thinning medication or if you have had a hemorrhagic stroke. Talk to your doctor about whether it is safe to drink alcohol while taking any medication.

**Focus on good nutrition.** This is an area you *do* have control over, so help yourself to avoid future strokes. If necessary, search out a nutritionist who can guide you with this. The Heart and Stroke Foundation website is also a great resource.

**Exercise within your limits.** Falls are a very real risk after a stroke, so walking with a buddy is a great idea.

**Stay positive and remain grateful.** Some days, you have to "fake it until you make it," especially in these first days. Keep trying to find the things and people you are grateful for. If you have a caregiver, express your awareness of their concern and care. If your caregiver is a family member or friend, remember they are learning about this new life with you.

**Find out about Group Long Term Disability.** It may be difficult to navigate forms at this point, so find help in obtaining and completing the paperwork necessary to initiate a claim for potential Long Term Disability benefits. In my case, we have a very efficient payroll/ benefits administrator at the Co-op office. She explained to me that for the first two weeks after my stroke I would receive sick leave benefits, so my paycheque wouldn't change. Eight days after my stroke, she helped me submit my claim. Our family physician was very quick to complete the Attending Physician's Statement.

On June 26th, I received a letter explaining my benefits would be retroactive back to June 5, and that my income would be 67 percent of my regular monthly salary. It also confirmed that payments would be made by direct deposit and that premiums would be waived for my portion of disability, basic life, and dental insurance through my group policy. It went on to say that my file would be reviewed for rehabilitation opportunities and that regular requests would be made to my doctor for updates on my progress.

It was almost two months since my last paycheque before I received my first, monthly disability payment. This financial strain added to my stress and anxiety.

**Use a file folder or some sort of storage container to keep paperwork** (such as all your reports, insurance applications, and notes from doctors' appointments) in one place. Don't worry about organizing it right away; hopefully that is a task you'll be able to manage down the road. It's so much easier to fill out the follow-up insurance forms when everything is in one place.

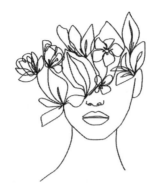

# Month 2
### (June 21–July 20, 2019)

## *June 22*

Blair left for British Columbia this morning with his parents and sister for a family trip they had been planning and looking forward to. I'm not feeling well enough for the long drive or the other demands of a trip. I'm still tired and finding that conversation drains my "brain battery." I often think of my brain in this way—as a battery, with some tasks draining it very quickly. I feel confident that I'll be okay home alone. After all, the stroke was a month ago. Jared and Justine will help me if I need them, and Blair will check in every day by phone. A week or so of guilt-free sleeping may be just what I need. I know that I'm the one putting pressure on myself to "get back to me." Blair has been a great caregiver, and he encourages me to let go of the office worries. I know it is what's best for me, but it's my "normal" that I'm really not ready to let go of.

## June 23

I drive to a neighbouring community fifteen minutes away to watch Justine play ball. This annual tournament is a great opportunity to cheer on local kids and to catch up with their parents, as well as to bring life to the bleachers. On my drive, I have a strange sensation that the ditches are moving by me much faster than the road is passing below me. This short trip is mentally exhausting. I'm trying to get more confident with driving so I can help with our planned trip to Ontario later this summer to attend my niece's wedding.

Justine's team wins the "A" side of the tournament. It's been a very exciting time, but I'm ready to go home and rest.

At home, and resting, I am missing Blair and realize I need to find something to fill my time while he is away. I have supplies for plastic canvas stitching, a craft I enjoyed immensely twenty-five years ago. I hope that the familiar task will be a good thing for me. I start by just making patterns on squares of canvas using different thread colours and stitching techniques. *Let's call them coasters,* I laugh to myself. Still, this simple project feels productive, familiar, and even relaxing—a great fit for me right now. I'm surprised that I can see a stitching error and not feel the need to tear everything out to correct it. I've always been a bit of a perfectionist. Is this part of the new me? I chuckle to myself that this new "perfectly imperfect" world may have to do for now.

## *June 24*

Another imperfection, however, was devastating: Earlier this month I had noticed that the toilet wasn't being flushed. I tried to not let my mind go to a dark place, but I couldn't help but wonder if Blair was okay. Early in his cancer journey, one of the oncologists mentioned that lung cancer is known to metastasize to the brain and we were to watch for the off-chance that Blair experiences headaches, personality changes, physical limitations, or behavioural changes. We were told that if we notice any of these changes, we should report them to our current oncologist. So, I thought, I'll keep an eye on him. *Please Lord, keep him safely in the palm of Your hand. Please heal his body, give him peace…bless both of us with peace, and Lord please give us Your wisdom to walk through this journey with grace and gratitude.*

Today, I see that the toilet again hasn't been flushed. But

Blair is gone. I realize that it's me! How am I forgetting to flush? I'm so embarrassed and at the same time relieved that this isn't a concerning symptom of Blair's cancer progressing. I want to cry. *Why hasn't Blair said something to me? What else am I forgetting?* He is so gracious at not making me feel any more "less than" I'm already feeling. "Less than" I was just over a month ago. *Lord, please keep me mindful of how much this man loves me. Thank you for his patience and compassion. Please bless him today and always.*

I am going to use the bathroom door and/or light switch as my memory cue. When I leave the bathroom and touch the light switch or door, I'll remember to check that I've flushed. I can do this. (*I had to very consciously go back and flush the toilet for a month or so before it became a habit again.*)

## June 25

I am driving to a friend's for coffee. The ditches are still moving way too fast.

I enjoy our visit and then I leave to meet Justine for lunch, just a thirty-minute drive away. I drive a short distance, and feel extreme fatigue setting in. Unsure that it's safe to carry on, I call her to cancel and I head back home. This is both frustrating and frightening. *Please Lord, get me home safely without hurting anyone along the way.* Once home, I immediately fall asleep, then wake to find I've slept for an hour and a half. It was the right decision to cancel for today. I worry, again: *Will this get better? How will this fatigue fit into my work life?*

## June 26

I'm determined to remain social, but I'm experiencing fear that I'm losing my ease around others. Faced with invitations, I often think that it would be so much easier to just stay home and rest. Today I visit some neighbours in our condo building, but I have to keep the visit short. It seems that even simple conversation makes my head tired. I head back home and stitch for a while—and then have another long nap.

## June 27

Blair is enjoying his trip with his family. They are visiting relatives they haven't seen in some time and sharing wonderful stories and memories. During today's check-in and conversation, Blair and I decide that the long drive to Ontario this summer is not a good idea and that we should fly instead. We want to be in good shape for my niece's wedding, which is the purpose of our visit. It will be so good to see my Ontario family and assure them I'm okay.

## *June 28*

At 8:30 a.m., a call from my younger brother startles me awake. He lives in Saskatchewan, but is visiting friends and family in Ontario and realized that he needs to have his licence plate renewed for the vehicle he's driving— ASAP. He asks if I can go to the insurance and licensing office and renew it before noon today.

During that call, my phone beeps with a Facebook private message; it's an urgent-sounding question regarding my home business in kitchenware sales. The customer wants information about a warranty, and I need to find the answer.

Too much! My brain is shutting down before I can deal with either of these requests.

I feel like I am in a state of waking, but yet not awake. I have a growing pressure in my head. I need to have a bath and wash my hair before I go out. Maybe I'll nap in the tub, I think.

Thirty minutes later, I still can't see straight. I can't focus my eyes to curl my hair or even watch the TV I turned on while getting ready. I don't know how to explain these visual disturbances other than to say it's like looking through a kaleidoscope and there is only a small, pinpoint area that allows me to see properly. I am feeling anxious about going out because I still can't see well.

The pressure in my head is more than a headache. (Reflecting on the situation later, I didn't seem to be able to reason that I might need medical attention. My sole focus was to get out and renew my brother's license plates.)

I'm too unsteady and my vision is too limited to walk safely to the office a few blocks away. I decide that taking the car is the safer option. I realize later that this was a bad and potentially dangerous decision, but at the time it felt safer.

I feel very emotional at the insurance office and break down in tears when one of the employees tells me about her cat that had been hit by a car and had to be put down. I'm actually not a fan of cats (to put it mildly, as anyone who knows me will attest) so while I would normally have been sympathetic, this more dramatic response was very unusual for me.

Maybe if I eat, I reason, my head will feel better. I head off to a local burger joint for a take-out meal. I'm back at home, and the burger tastes very bitter. I lie down for a rest. When I awaken, it's two hours later. Still not feeling well, I try another nap. After fifteen minutes of sleep, I feel much better.

Friends have invited me out for supper, and I'm actually feeling well enough to join them. What a bizarre day. I definitely made some bad choices. If Blair were home he would have run the errand. Now I wonder: *Can I trust my own judgement?*

I think that by now my unsteadiness should have resolved, and I decide I need a physiotherapist. Nobody has referred me to one, so I decide I will use my connections at the local hospital and try to self-refer.

## June 30

Blair is home from his trip! I'm so relieved to have him here to hold and to talk to and also to monitor my decisions. I missed my best friend's presence. I am so tired, but at least I am sleeping well with Blair back home.

## July 1

I am happily sitting with a friend in the sunshine, awaiting the Canada Day parade. Almost unconsciously, but beneficially, I am sitting at the end of a long row of camp chairs. It's a bit quieter here, with fewer people to talk to, but I am glad to be taking part in the celebration, and I feel safe.

Our small town of Assiniboia, population approximately 2400, has great community spirit. Volunteers with *Communities in Bloom* make sure that all our public spaces have beautiful flower gardens and pots, making Main Street colourful and welcoming. As we wait for the parade to begin, we admire the flowering pots just down the block.

There's something about living in small-town Saskatchewan that brings me great comfort and peace. Familiar faces, friendly greetings, and the slower pace of life that encourages a social attitude of taking time to stop. Truly, it's where everyone knows your name. For the most part, that's an asset to small-town living.

Several people stop to say hello as they line up their chairs along the sidewalk. I enjoy the excited anticipation in the air and the warm sun on my skin.

Here it comes, the siren of the police car that leads the way. The children near us are overjoyed with excitement from the flashing lights and loud noises. I brace myself for the swirl of imbalance the volume of the siren evokes. It passes quickly once the siren stops.

I don't know all the children riding their bikes in the parade and along the parade route, but I can pick out some family resemblances that are identifiable after living in and around the community for decades.

We wave at the people in the parade and admire their work—some floats have bright colours and flashing lights, some have themes, some have music playing. It's good to be outside and feel a part of the community again. I've been mostly staying inside, where I feel safest, for some time.

As the Member Relations Officer for the Co-op, part of my job was to make sure we had a float for the July 1st parade in the summer and the Parade of Lights in the winter. It's always fun to see how creative the residents and businesses can be. I experience a small ache in my heart when I see the Co-op float go by and know that I had no part in it. I really enjoyed that task—the creative process of taking float suggestions from team members and then watching the vision come to life for our public unveiling. For the last few summers, our larger, umbrella company, Federated Co-op Limited (FCL), has created summer floats that could be rented and assembled, and they have a very professional look. That is the float that is in this parade. I had eagerly watched and waited to see what it would look like.

The parade lasts nearly thirty minutes, and the fire truck brings up the rear, its siren signaling the end.

People don't rush to leave their chairs along the sidewalk. They opt to stay and visit a bit, commenting on the many floats.

We have a wonderful Recreation and Community Wellness co-ordinator in Assiniboia, and she has many activities planned for the day. The children tug on the adults, encouraging them, not so gently, to move on to the next event.

I'm overwhelmed. The noise and all the visual stimulation have tired my brain. I go home to nap and happily fall into sleep.

Later, I am energized enough for a 2.3-km walk with Blair. I can walk distances with someone by my side but feel too off balance when walking alone. I wonder sometimes if this is psychological. The massage therapist in me thinks that my proprioceptors aren't responding appropriately. These are the sensory receptors on the nerve endings of the inner ear, muscles, skin, joints, tendons, and other tissues, and they facilitate a coordinated neurological and physiological response to body movement. I'm not sure that this is part of my problem, but it's worth thinking about and following up on with the physiotherapist.

## *July 2*

Blair and I are driving to Moose Jaw for his dental appointment. As it happens, we have time to go on to Regina for me to go to a craft-supply store to stock up on my plastic canvas supplies. I'm becoming much more creative with my projects, and I feel good about accomplishing them. I'm excited to go into the store. Blair has an errand to run, so he drops me off.

Almost immediately on entering the big store I feel my head start to spin. I focus on heading to where I think my items are located. I feel terrible. I stop at the yarn section and just stare at some pastel-coloured yarns, trying to regain focus until I feel well enough to move on. It doesn't even occur to me to adjust my posture to see if that will help. During massage training, I learned the importance of posture. In fact, one of our goals as a RMT (Registered Massage Therapist) is to help relax or strengthen muscles to allow ideal alignment of ears over shoulders over hips over ankles. Proper posture improves balance, improves breathing, relieves back pain, improves circulation and digestion, and even helps improve concentration. I know all of this. Now to be aware of my posture and consciously make adjustments as needed.

As soon as I leave that section of the store, I feel like I'm going to lose control of my bowels. I text Blair to come back to get me. As soon as I leave the building, I feel better. I did not get what I went in for.

It feels strange and sad to have such an adverse reaction to what I was expecting to be an exciting and pleasurable outing. The visual and aural stimulation of a store—the array of colours, music, loudspeaker announcements, other shoppers—it's all too much.

I wish someone had told me to expect this. I wish I knew what was happening, physiologically. *Is this normal for people who have had a stroke?* I had no answers.

## *July 3*

The morning started with a phone call that was unsettling. It didn't wake me, and it was only about a change to an appointment date, but it was a disruption to how I thought our day would start, and I found it stressful. We are now off to see Blair's folks for lunch, and I plan to meet a friend later in the afternoon. But I am feeling an increased level of brain fog today. I am worried, because having too many events in a day is taxing mentally. Now I have a headache and pressure in my head.

I wonder if my friends and relatives have a sense of how hard this is sometimes. When I feel my energy dropping,

I get very quiet, and hope that I don't fall asleep. Do they know that? Or is my quietness interpreted as being aloof or moody? I want to explain, but when I do my words sound to me like poor excuses and I don't even want to hear myself say them anymore.

## *July 5*

Blair and I are driving to Medicine Hat, Alberta, for a friend's wedding. I drive for about thirty minutes and then immediately sleep for over an hour while Blair takes over the wheel.

## *July 6*

This morning I woke up with bruises on my arm and left breast. No idea where they came from. I try to reason that I've been on blood thinners for a month and a half and that possibly I've met a certain saturation rate. I won't panic. But this is an example of things that are happening to me without me expecting them and without me understanding them. These unknowns are stressful and sometimes frightening.

My friend's wedding is beautiful. I am enjoy talking with some hometown friends who are also attending. I push through fatigue as the day goes on.

I develop a persistent headache while trying to fall sleep. These nighttime headaches are happening more often, especially on days when I push myself beyond the feeling that it's time to rest.

It felt good to dress up and feel beautiful. *Did I look confident? Did I convince everyone that this fatigue and these headaches are manageable?*

## *July 9*

I am beginning to feel more confident in walking alone.

I'm also driving a short distance today, with Blair in the passenger's seat. I feel much more confident when Blair is with me, but I'm trying to be more independent. We are on our way to a family gathering for my in-laws' wedding anniversary.

Justine passed her final Pharmacy Licensing Exam! I'm so proud of her. She landed a job shortly after graduation (pharmacy grads in Saskatchewan work with a conditional licence until completing the final exam). I've always felt that she's proud of me and of my academic and volunteer accomplishments. I know she's still proud of me, but the weight of her worrying about me is showing. With her school pressures, her dad's cancer, and my stroke, she's had a lot of extra concerns. I sense that her anxiety is increasing, but she is always solicitous and so considerate of me.

Jared is also incredibly affectionate. I love feeling his long, strong arms when they wrap me in a hug. I've lately been feeling some sadness and guilt about him, because of his struggles in school. I know that I expected too much from him. In Kindergarten, he had a bad fall off his bike— so severe that it broke his helmet. We took him to the ER, and he was checked out and treated for abrasions. Now, looking back, and with my new awareness of brain injury, I suspect that he may have suffered some brain trauma. I have a new respect for how hard he's worked all these years to maintain concentration and try to meet my expectation of better grades. I tell him that. He hugs me and says, "Welcome to my world." I know he says it with great love and understanding. I want to hug the little boy in him whom I pushed to work harder and do better at school.

## July 10

Today is my first physio assessment! I am at Moose Jaw hospital. Testing shows a right-side weakness. We are scheduling a regular exercise program at our local hospital, to start next week. Yay! It finally feels like something is being done to help me get back on track and to feel more stable walking.

I'm also making an appointment to see an occupational therapist, with a referral from my physiotherapist. I'm so happy to feel that I'm receiving support. I suddenly don't feel so alone.

Until now, I feel like I have been freefalling and trying to take hold of the safety net before I fall too far to be fixed.

The physiotherapist is providing me with great written information on strokes. Even though reading causes me extreme headaches, and my comprehension seems to be limited, I'm happy to have something in hand that I can learn from. *Why didn't this happen sooner?* I ask myself.

## *July 11*

Justine has a shift as the relief pharmacist in a community ninety minutes away so I have come along to spend a couple days with her and have a change of scenery. I had planned to stitch in the hotel room while she works, but I feel very nauseous today. I'm not sure what that is about; nausea has not been usual, despite all my dizziness.

## *July 12*

We plan to head home after Justine's last shift. I am overwhelmed by all I have to do to pack up and check out of the hotel room by 1 p.m. I experience head pressure and visual impairment so severe I can't even watch TV or stitch. I go back to bed to sleep. Justine arrives at one to pick me up, but even after four hours of sleep, I still feel unwell. I had planned to shop until Justine is done her shift at five.

I have always enjoyed the adventure of shopping, looking for those unique items that would work to solve a problem or add interest to my wardrobe or home space. It is fun to discover new stores and boutiques. I have seen a few worth investigating. I decide to push past feeling unwell and step into a store, maybe even just to distract me from my current state of mind.

It didn't work. The visual stimulation makes me feel off balance. My stomach is sensitive to the smells. The normally calming music, played to make the shopping experience more pleasurable is adding to a now intensifying headache. I know I have to leave and save this adventure for another day.

I find a shady tree to park under and sleep until it's time to pick her up. As Justine drives home, I sleep. I wake up at six and feel well for the first time today. We had such a short time to visit, but I enjoyed every minute of being with her.

## *July 13*

I am feeling steadier with my physio exercises. Standing on my right leg, I am almost as steady as on my left. Progress! I am so grateful for that measurable improvement.

## *July 15*

Late at night, I am awake and praying desperately for confirmation that God is taking care of our finances. Why do worries feel so intense at night?

I'm missing playing cards with friends. We played canasta almost weekly on Wednesday afternoons, on my day off. A friend is over for some "card therapy" today. We're playing a few hands to see what I can manage. I enjoy the mental game of playing and it feels good to be stimulating that part of my brain again, but I am so tired. I feel some confusion but mostly just fatigue. It was so worth it though, just to connect with friends.

The biggest adjustments for me, I realize, are not being able to make quick, critical-thinking decisions and the lack of ability to read for enjoyment. I am just trusting and hoping that this is temporary.

## July 16

Today my physio exercise program starts at the local hospital. My oxygen saturation rate ($O_2$) is low at 92 percent, I am told. Again, I am not sure why.

We are leaving next week for Ontario so we need to start packing. Just thinking about what needs to go in the suitcase is as exhausting as any physical activity. Will I forget something? Possibly. Will it be the end of the world? No. Again, I smile at the thought of the ease that I am accepting living in a perfectly imperfect world.

## July 17

Today is my 61st birthday. I've been cleared for having a massage (more than six weeks has passed since my surgery) so this morning I am enjoying that time of self-care. I go home for a nap before joining my in-laws for a birthday lunch. I feel like I do a pretty good job of keeping up the smiles during lunch. I'm getting better at staying engaged without speaking so I can at least portray the illusion that I'm better.

## July 18

I have an appointment with my family physician. Two months have passed since my stroke. The doctor is not concerned about my O$_2$ level when I tell him about it. He is referring me to our local Stroke Prevention Clinic at my request. I still want to know why I had the stroke when I had no risk factors. My doctor is recommending another three to six months off work. I'm still getting headaches and visual disturbances, and I struggle to multi-task. Although I was hoping to be back to work sooner than this, I'm definitely not feeling like I could perform my work tasks well enough.

Today is also my appointment with an occupational therapist (OT). She explains that this is her last day of working down in our area and a replacement OT hasn't been hired yet. She confirms that tasks like puzzles and handwork are wonderful to keep one's thoughts in the present and avoid worrying about the future. After hearing my many thoughts and concerns, she suggests that I slow down, spend less time on the computer, and try not to read—to allow my brain to rest and heal. She encourages napping as needed and to relax. She reminds me that I have insurance so I should try not to panic about finances right now. She says I'll get back to work when I'm ready.

I understand all this on an intellectual level, but emotionally I'm in a panic state and don't want to let go of my life as it was a few months ago. I want to quickly get back to the way I was. I want to enjoy reading without having to constantly reread because my comprehension isn't what it used to be. And I'm tired of being a burden!

I share this with her: it's been two months and I'm feeling a little more confident being out of the house. I have no obvious physical impairments, so people assume I've recovered and am ready to go back to work. "You look good," they often say. I totally understand how it might appear that I'm healed. But deep down, with limited filters, I want to scream that I can try to make myself look good, I can still put on my makeup, but I'm sure not healed. I know I should simply explain this to people, but it's a situation so emotionally fraught that I'm afraid to even comment for fear of having a meltdown. A smile and nod is as much as I can offer right now. This therapist is wonderful. She makes me feel heard. My soul has some comfort in being able to share, and unload, all of this with her.

She gives me a Mini-Mental State Exam (MMSE) and begins a cognitive assessment, but I can feel my brain crashing and fatigue coming on, so we don't finish it.

As the appointment winds down, she reminds me that I have no insurance coverage if I have an accident while driving my vehicle. With our provincial vehicle insurance, there is no coverage for six months after a stroke.

*What?????* It's been two months, and this is the first I've heard of this. I have driven very infrequently and have been safe, but I would never have put myself behind the wheel if I'd known this. My administrative mind wonders how this information was not made available to me sooner. How did this fall through the cracks? I'm back to anger and frustration!

## *July 19*

I am feeling that I need more purpose to my days. Blair was asked if he would volunteer to tend bar at the local Polkafest tonight for two hours. So I'm volunteering with him. It's not very busy on this 7–9 p.m. shift, so the pace is perfect. The lighting is low and the music is not too loud. I am enjoying the music and watching the dancers. It's so good to feel useful.

## *July 20, 2019*

Today we are travelling with Blair's mom and dad for a family birthday and anniversary celebration four hours away. I sleep on the drive there. Although I'm enjoying seeing everyone, after a few hours I'm heading to the car to sleep until everyone is ready to leave. Sometimes I can fake it and sometimes the fatigue wins. I'm thankful that my family is being understanding. I feel bad leaving, and awkward too. I hope they know I'm trying to make an effort to fit back into our social world.

## *What I have learned ...*

**Be kind to yourself and allow yourself time to heal.** Take time to rest. Especially for those with cognitive rather than physical impairments, it's hard to not push to get back to "normal." Trust that others who have experienced this have taken a year or more to heal. I know you want to be the exception to that rule. I did.

**Limit screen time.** At this point in your recovery, you may be bored and want to entertain yourself with video games or checking out your social media. May I suggest a healthier option as suggested to me by the occupational therapist—working on picture puzzles and or handcrafts will not only fill your days, it will keep you from worrying about the future.

Why is it hard on our head to be on a computer screen? According to the Brain Injury Society of Toronto: [1]

- Images that appear on LCD screens are made up of pixels that refresh at a rate of 60 times per second even when the content on the screen is not changing.
- The rapid movement of these pixels means that when we look at screens for too long, we strain our eye muscles.

53

- For someone who has suffered a brain injury, this strain can be detrimental.
- The backlighting of LCD screens can cause cognitive fatigue, headaches, dizziness, and nausea in brain-injured patients.

**Reach out to your local chapter of the Brain Injury Association.** In Canada, you can find your closest chapter at: www.braininjurycanada.ca. I often felt that my recovery was my mountain to climb alone. Please know that there is great support through both the provincial chapters and Brain Injury Canada. You'll have an opportunity to meet others with acquired brain injuries and ask questions that make sense to someone else. It is also a great resource for your caregiver to be able to understand what it's like to live with a brain injury.

**Find out about your insurance coverage.** You've probably already started applying for and maybe even receiving some group benefits through work. I was surprised to find that, because I was over the age of sixty when my stroke occurred, I only had twelve months of long-term disability coverage. Had I been under the age of sixty, my coverage would have been twenty-four months. Insurance coverage varies dramatically with different companies' policies. For example, with my husband's cancer, he has long-term disability benefits until age sixty-five.

At month two, I wasn't able to cognitively work through these policy details, but hopefully your caregiver or someone you trust will be able to help you.

Do you have disability insurance coverage on:

- Your line of credit at the bank?
- Your credit card?
- Your life insurance policies through a waiver of premium rider?

Do you have a critical illness insurance policy? Does it cover stroke?

Canada Pension Plan Disability coverage has a four-month waiting period which we will discuss in "What I have learned ..." in chapter four.

**Cognitive Assessment.** This is an assessment tool completed by occupational therapists, psychiatrists, or neurologists to make a diagnosis and understand a patient's cognitive capabilities. It includes a series of questions and tasks designed to help measure mental functions such as memory, language, and the ability to recognize objects. Some insurance companies require this in order to approve your claim, to determine that you have a cognitive impairment lasting more than thirty days. This is an assessment that should take place in month two of recovery.

**You are doing fine!** It will take time, but it will get better. Be sure to journal your struggles and successes so you can see how far you've come as time passes.

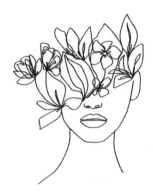

## Month 3

(July 21–August 20, 2019)

### *July 22*

I checked with my insurance company to see if leaving the province would affect my disability insurance income. The representative said that if my family physician deems me well enough to fly, the company has no concerns. Our family doctor has approved our flying to Ontario. I'm elated! On July 24 we will be on our way.

We are still waiting for my long-term disability insurers to start depositing monthly payments. Coverage has been approved until June 2020. Because I was older than sixty when the stroke occurred, I have coverage for only one year. I have already surpassed the one-month waiting period.

## *July 23*

In Regina, I have my follow-up appointment with the surgeon. He says that the incision looks good. He will book a follow-up carotid ultrasound for five months post-surgery. I have a chance to ask the surgeon about something that has been causing me a lot of anxiety: Could there be plaque in my heart? He says that happens in only 10 percent of the cases in which plaque is found in the carotid arteries. This news comes as a great relief to me. I also mention that my $O_2$ (oxygen) saturation rate remains at about 92. He suggests that we continue to monitor that. Ninety-five or higher is a more normal level.

Another question I have for the surgeon is about my handwriting. It has changed considerably, and sometimes I find it hard to remember spelling and proper word choices. I ask if that is normal and whether it will improve. He says that when speech is affected, those skills are also often affected. I found this both interesting and concerning. The doctor explains that there is no indication whether this will improve.

He goes on to tell me that my symptoms are consistent

with someone who is recovering from a concussion. He says that the stroke was a brain injury, and then the surgery—although it was on my neck—affected blood flow to the brain and was also an assault considered to be a brain injury. These two injuries, plus an earlier brain injury I had in 1975, when I was in a car accident and suffered a blow to the head, will all affect the rate at which I recover.

From the time I was a fifteen-year-old girl, then living in rural southwestern Ontario, I would travel every summer to a very small Saskatchewan community south of Assiniboia to help a family who were once neighbours of my family in Ontario—they had lived across the gravel road from us. While visiting, I would help with their foster children. Back in the early '70s, I'd jump on the train and enjoy the fifty-hour journey to Saskatchewan. It was a different time then. I never felt unsafe. Being the middle child of five children, I could hardly wait to just sit on the train and read or people-watch. The first summer I made the journey, many young people were heading to British Columbia to work as tree planters. That was a wonderful trip, as some fellow passengers were musicians and they entertained us for hours. I loved it! When the train would fall quiet, I'd turn on my overhead light and read until I fell asleep. I felt as though I'd been living a great adventure. Travel has always appeared to me.

The year I was turning seventeen, I told my mother that I wanted to take my Grade 12 year in Saskatchewan and live with the family I'd stayed with during my western visits. She agreed. My two older siblings were done school by then. I had made many good friends in Saskatchewan and I saw this as something I just really wanted to do— another adventure.

On September 25, 1975, I went to a wedding cabaret in a very rural, remote area of Saskatchewan. In those days, the cabarets were open to the whole community to come and celebrate with the happy couple. After the cabaret ended that September day, we were invited to the bride's family farm to continue the celebrating.

I don't remember the wedding. I don't remember the accident. I can't even remember most of the year prior to the accident. I'm not sure if I have ever had real memories of the accident or if I am simply familiar with the stories that were told about that night, terrifying in retrospect.

The story is that three friends and I left the party at the farm, the four of us in the truck. It was before the days of mandatory seat belts. We came to a T in the road. There was no sign to indicate that the road ended. We flew over the highway and hit a dirt bank. The other three occupants were thrown out of the vehicle, but I was pinned in. We later heard that there were indentations in the dash where our heads had hit.

There was no local ambulance service back then, so we waited for the ambulance to arrive from Regina, which was nearly a three-hour drive from the accident site. We were blessed to have a local registered nurse and her husband come across the accident first. Without a doubt she was our angel.

We all survived. Everyone had injuries, of varying degrees. I had a broken leg and a broken nose, I bit my lower lip in half, and I lost a front tooth. I also had a severe head injury. I wouldn't wake for five days after the accident.

I do have bits and pieces of memories of this time. I have a memory of waking in the hospital, confused, and feeling that the lights were too bright. I had a headache. I saw a small table beside the bed, with a drawer. I must have thought that the drawer held answers because I remember wanting to open it to find out where I was, what happened, and why I hurt. When I did open it, I found all my bloody clothes. I recognized my maroon-coloured pants and bloodied white shirt. The old blood had a distinct odour. I was shocked and confused.

I tried to sit, to get my bearings. This nauseated me. A nurse came into the room and looked happy to see me awake. I knew I was going to vomit. She must have sensed what was going on and handed me a kidney dish. I vomited such large blood clots that I struggled to breathe as they were coming up from my stomach. My broken nose was packed with gauze so the only means of getting oxygen was through my mouth. I was frightened. My brain was sluggish.

I knew I was in the hospital on my own. I knew that my parents were in Ontario and that my mom was opening her new restaurant on the weekend, so I couldn't expect her to come get me. Times were different then, and children were more independent and self-reliant, at least in my experience; this was in the days before cellphones, video calls, or messaging. Long-distance calls were very expensive and interprovincial travel was uncommon. So I was pretty much on my own.

Years later, I read my mom's diary of the days surrounding my accident. She was just told by the couple that I was staying with that I'd been in a car accident and had only broken my arm—which I hadn't.

I stayed in hospital for nearly two weeks. I had many episodes of vomiting blood. They eventually found that I had a bleed in my brain cavity or sinuses. I had surgery to repair the bleeding structures and was finally released back to the care of the family I was staying with.

My recovery was slow. My leg was in a cast longer than the usual six or eight weeks, but I don't remember how long. A local schoolteacher picked me up every day for school so I didn't have to try to climb the steps of the bus. It was the spring of 1976, six months after the accident, before I had surgery to realign my broken nose. It was also around that time when I received the dental work to replace the gap in my smile.

I still experience incredible anxiety when I hear gravel hitting the underside of any vehicle I'm riding in. I know that blood in my mouth makes me feel like I'm going into shock, so when I had to have my wisdom teeth removed, I was sedated. Also, and somewhat oddly, Elton John's song "Someone Saved My Life Tonight" still shakes me to the core. I remember a doctor once telling me that perhaps that song was playing either when the accident happened or when I became conscious. Even though the song haunts me, the words make me think, with so much gratitude, of the nurse who was first to come across our accident.

I remember how hard school was that year, how hard it was for me to learn. I was never an A student—a B or C student at best. That year I just barely passed my classes. But I did pass, and I graduated with the rest of the class. It was such a celebration, such a feeling of accomplishment.

After that year of brain fog following the accident, I started to find that learning came more easily to me and I craved new information. A friend even told me that I had an affinity for learning. She was right. I had a feeling, or realization, that there is so much that I know I don't know, and I wanted to understand more.

After high school, I returned to Ontario to work for my dad at his farm implement dealership. After about a year, I realized how much I missed my friends and life back in Saskatchewan. So, I headed back.

My newfound ease with studying and learning manifested in my taking a series of courses and making varied career moves. I so enjoyed the feeling of soaking up new knowledge and skills.

Two years after high school, I took a one-year office education course in Moose Jaw. Following that success, I took advanced training at my administration job with a life insurance company and received the designation Fellow of the Life Management Institute (FLMI) with a specialty in Selection of Risk and Information Systems (that's what they called computer training before computers were commonplace in offices). I went on to study medical terminology and eventually got a job as a receptionist at a doctor's office. While there, I trained as a Medical Records Technician (now called a Health Information

Manager). I further trained as a Chartered Herbalist and a Registered Massage Therapist (RMT). Finally, I followed a new interest in Credit Training where I earned a certificate in Commercial Credit Administration, just before my stroke.

Now, I feel like I'm mourning the loss of my ability to read and comprehend. I seem to be able to conduct a Google search but before I can find the answer to my question my head begins to ache and my eyes create the odd shapes that cloud my vision. I read and reread, wanting the words to sink in, to make sense, to show me the answer I'm looking for. I'm so frustrated! I want to be able to figure out how to fix the residual effects of my stroke. What exercises or therapies can I use to help myself? What has research shown on recovery rates? Is it expected that my cognitive abilities will return? Will I be able to learn again? Read for pure enjoyment?

## *July 24*

I am excited for our flight to Ontario for my niece's wedding. It brings back memories of the excitement of travel that I felt as a youth.

We have a layover in Winnipeg, so we decide to spend some time in the lounge. My phone keeps beeping. Oh no! It's WestJet, paging Blair. We rush to the gate as they announce, "Final call for Blair and Julianne Heagy. Final call for Blair and Julianne Heagy." Darn it! I thought I had planned everything so well, but, again, I was confused by numbers. I was sure we had two hours between flights.

On board, I feel so relieved that we made the flight. I forget that I can't always trust my interpretation of numbers. Blair is so used to me taking the lead in our travel plans that he didn't question it either. We are both learning to navigate our new roles in this post-stroke world.

## *July 27*

A beautiful day for a wedding. The outdoor, country setting is so relaxing. The venue isn't far from London, where we're staying, so we're already gauging how much time we will need to plan for our return to our rented accommodations. Our niece is such a beautiful bride and she has a handsome groom. My brother is so proud of his daughter. You can see it in the way he looks at her. She is the first of her generation to get married. I think of my older sister who passed away in 2009 of breast cancer, and deeply wish she could be with us for our niece's wedding. I think about how proud she would have been to see her granddaughters all dressed up and looking gorgeous and happy today.

The cousins are all enjoying their time together. What a wonderful reason to dress up and dance. My heart is full and happy. Blair and I love to dance, and are good at it, I have to say. When I pause to think about our reality, I realize we make quite a pair: I am imbalanced from a stroke, and he has reduced lung capacity from his illness. But we still do what we can to slip into a good old two-step or a waltz. We dance with each other compassionately as I try to anticipate when his breath is too laboured, and he holds me close to help me fight the imbalance when moving through quick steps and turns. We don't last long past the supper and dance, but we are so happy that we were able to attend.

## *August 1*

We had planned to fly home the day after the wedding, but our family had received a call letting us know that there was a long-term care bed available for Dad, in London, about half an hour's drive from his home. He needed a higher level of care due to medical concerns. He was also needing support in case of a fall, preparation of meals, laundry service, and general personal care. Blair and I wanted to stay and help with packing up Dad's apartment and visit him in his new home, with the hope of helping him to settle in. It was an emotional time for Dad. He took some convincing to leave his current home.

My brother and sister had tried to encourage Dad to just go and look at the room that had been offered to him. He would seem agreeable, but when the time came to pick him up, he said he was content to stay where he was. Nobody wanted to force him to go, but we all knew it would be the safest move for him. At one point, we three siblings were outside of Dad's apartment discussing how to proceed. What would we do if he was adamant about not moving? Blair was with Dad inside. In his gentle manner, Blair calmly suggested to Dad that it wouldn't hurt to just go have a look. By the time we went back in, Dad had agreed to make the trip to London to see where he'd be staying.

He did make the move, and we were grateful, both for his well-being and also because it took some pressure off my sister and brother, as they were sharing the responsibility of Dad's caregiving.

There was a lot to do to empty and clean Dad's apartment. Although I knew I needed to rest, I was so happy to be able to give a hand. Living so far away from my family, I often missed out on the routine of their lives. It was good to be able to help. I knew I'd rest when I got home.

## *August 5*

We have an uneventful return flight home—no mad dash

to the gate, now that we are aware that I need Blair's help in watching the clock and locating gate numbers. It was such a good visit, although it was emotionally difficult to move Dad. I also came to the conclusion that I'm not very comfortable travelling right now, and will probably not be too eager to book another trip anywhere for a while. My confidence has definitely been shaken.

## *August 7*

Safely back home in Assiniboia. The co-worker who was helping to keep the paper moving on my desk at the Co-op needs some information about a donation I had approved. I can't remember how the donation had been handled, so I say that I'll come in and check my files. It will be easy for me to find the answer, I assure my workmate. All I have to do is simply pull the file and find the answer in my notes.

In my office, it feels good to be sitting at my desk and to see my workmates and assure them I was starting to see some minor improvements. After some chatting and updating, I decide I'd better get to the task at hand, feeling confident that I know exactly where to find the answer to the question. But I can't figure out how to find the file. This is so frustrating! My filing system is so easy to use—it is so logically ordered. I rifle through files and papers, hoping my system would come to me, that it would make sense. I am trying not to panic. Now I'm in tears and embarrassed. I have to tell my co-worker that I can't figure it out. I feel so frustrated and annoyed. This should have been so easy! She assures me it's okay.

As I leave, I feel completely defeated, lowering my head to avoid eye contact with anyone I might meet in the hallway. And now I need to negotiate those damn stairs down to the main level. I just want to get out of here! This is the day I know that I won't be coming back soon. I realize I've been in denial about how much the stroke has affected me.

Lately I've been frustrated with well-meaning family, friends, and acquaintances who still say, "You're looking good. Back to work?" Some days I want to scream, "I always try to look good! But I'm not!" I'm glad I'm able to stop myself from saying this out loud. My filter against saying inappropriate things isn't as good as it used to be.

My internal dialogue responds, No, I'm not back to work. I struggle to read, and I can't look at a computer screen very long. I can't trust myself with numbers. My balance comes and goes, and I am extremely fatigued much of the time. So no, I'm not back to work!

I'm still surprised at how many people don't know I've had a stroke. I appreciate that the administration and management staff at work have respected my privacy. However, I wonder what the other staff, and customers, think? Do they think I'm on an extended holiday? Do they think Blair's health has taken a turn for the worse? Do they think I've been fired from, or have left, the Co-op?

Sometimes I meet people who know about my stroke yet don't ask how I'm doing. Instead, they ask about Blair. He's been battling cancer for six years now and amazes us all with his positive attitude and how he's managed to beat all the odds. On one hand, I sincerely appreciate their interest and concern for him. On the other hand, I feel invisible. Sadly, it makes me feel that I don't matter. Maybe that's why I'm feeling more sensitive to fielding these questions about Blair and not me. Is this selfish? Does this make me a bad person?

## *August 7–9*

Justine had suggested that she and I go for a little getaway to just rest and relax. We have booked a few nights near Saco, Montana, where there is a small resort with hot springs. I've heard of Saco but have never been here. I thought it was much farther away than it actually is, and we arrive in under two hours. What a fun little western spot! We enjoy the mineral water in the pool. We spend the rest of our time binge-watching "Nurse Jackie" while

I work on a plastic canvas project.

I feel that I'm not the strong mom Justine has been proud of in the past. I am feeling more like a burden—and I am not loving this feeling. I sense that she thinks she has to entertain me, watch over me, guide me. Even though I really enjoy our time together, I wish I could take some of the weight off her shoulders. I'm not ready for her to be my caregiver.

## *August 12*

A representative of my group insurance company calls to check on my progress. He is very kind and empathetic. I tell him how frustrated I am with my progress. I tell him about the disappointing visit to my office where I couldn't make sense of the files. I'm happy to report to him that I've started some physio exercises and am hoping that my balance will start to improve. He was very encouraging and said it's not unheard of to need the full year to get back on track. I think to myself, Maybe for others but not for me! I tell him I'm trying to do some computer work to keep up my skills but find that the headaches make this really hard. He suggests that I give my brain a rest. He strongly suggests that I stop trying to work on the computer and try not to read—to let my brain heal. I am grateful for his understanding; I had been worried that I would be pressured to be better.

## *August 12 - 19*

I am at my physio session at our local hospital. It feels good to be doing physical activity safely. I spin twenty minutes on a lateral recumbent bike and do some balancing exercises. I feel safe on the bike. The balancing exercises are done with the use of rails on either side of me, like the parallel bars in our gym class back in high school, but lower. This too feels safe, and with each session I feel more confident. I can last twenty to thirty seconds while standing on one foot before I need to grab the rails. As I attend more appointments, I try things like standing on one foot with my eyes closed or with my head turned to the left or right. I'm working up to standing on an uneven surface like a pillow to fire up my proprioceptors that help with balance.

I like to practise these exercises at home in the kitchen while I'm cooking. The counter and the island are all within close range, so grabbing hold of a solid surface is easily done. I'm finding the balancing exercises more tiring than the physical exercises, but I appreciate that they are something I can do, something I can control to help me recover.

## *August 20*

Today I receive a massage. I am so close to tears.

Throughout the appointment, I hope that I can just keep it together, and also hope that the massage will help settle me down. My massage therapist, who is also a friend, is so very professional. She provides a safe place, and our time together is very quiet. She accepts my stifled sobs. I'm still feeling so overwhelmed by my slow progress, our financial situation, my frustrations with not being able to read or learn. I just want this to get better!

Lately, I've been even more concerned about our finances. I know we are in better shape now than six years ago when Blair was first diagnosed with lung cancer. He was the Plant Manager at a local certified grain-cleaning plant and I was a full-time Registered Massage Therapist. I was also working part-time at our local hospital in the admitting and discharge department. When we were thrown into the whirlwind life that a cancer diagnosis demands, we found ourselves spending our 25th wedding anniversary in Blair's pre-op appointment to plan for the removal of the right upper lobe of his lung. Things seemed to happen very quickly after that. He had surgery, recovery, and chemotherapy, with a nearly two-hour travel time each way, for every appointment and treatment. For six months we were able to sleep in our own bed only a few times for more than one night. This meant that I was unable to keep up with my massage business. My massage clinic was in our home, and when we were home it was important to keep the house quiet so Blair could sleep.

With any insurance, the initial processing of a disability claim takes a few months. Blair's claim was no different. We had bills piling up and our bank account was empty. I had to make a few hard phone calls to the utility companies and others explaining that we would catch up our account when some money started coming in but we just couldn't pay right now. For the most part, our creditors were more than accommodating and assured us that an extension on our bills wouldn't affect our credit rating. I hadn't even considered that our credit rating would suffer from our inability to keep our payments current. That just added to my stress.

We had planned for our retirement. We had saved and prioritized. We were financially on track—until we weren't. What a helpless feeling. Our community held a fundraiser for us. We struggled with accepting their offer to help but finally gave in. Back then, I was the president of the Massage Therapist Association of Saskatchewan, and the board of directors had offered to pay for four nights' accommodation while we were in the city for treatments. We were—and still are—deeply grateful for these kindnesses.

Eventually, we had to draw from our investments just to keep up with the bills. Our retirement fund was shrinking.

We had a bit of a financial reprieve when Blair and I

were both able to return to work. A few years later, Blair's cancer returned and his left lower lobe had to be removed. He was deemed to have stage IV lung cancer and again his prognosis was poor. Clearly it was a tough go emotionally, but also financially. Blair was receiving a disability income that was a percentage of his regular income. I had to work fewer days so I could be there for Blair. Again our retirement fund took a hit. Emotionally exhausted, we relied heavily on a financial advisor to help us through this struggle. She reviewed our situation and, delicately, advised that our line of credit had life insurance coverage on Blair. She was very tactful at not letting our conversations get too dark when she recommended that we tap into our large, unused portion of the line of credit. That allowed us to breathe a bit. It was a financial cushion we hadn't thought of. During the following many meetings, she suggested that if Blair had a bucket list, this would be the place to find the funds to make sure we could check items off the list. It made sense at the time, and I absolutely wanted him to live all his dreams while we could.

As the balance of the line of credit increased so did the payments on it. We were managing fine though. I had a few extra jobs, so if it felt we were getting behind I'd take extra shifts or amp up sales with my home business selling kitchen tools and equipment. I've always been that way. If we ever wanted a trip or to upgrade a vehicle, I'd take on another short-term job or work more hours at the hospital. I didn't realize how much I relied on this extra income until I didn't have the ability to earn it.

I'm anxious over our finances as I don't have a plan or an opportunity to keep us caught up. All I can envision right now is that our retirement savings are going to continue to dwindle.

On top of this, many of our friends and relatives are preparing to, or have recently, retired. They are so pleased with their retirement incomes and by how much they are enjoying being home and letting the cheques roll in. Will that ever be us?

As I look back over the past three months since my stroke, I note I'm still sleeping a lot, feeling off-balance, and experiencing kaleidoscope-like visual disturbances—all after relatively minor mental tasks. I am definitely unable to multi-task. Blair knows that when my hand goes up I can't take in another question or thought. I can process only what I'm currently working on. This works very well for us but isn't received well or understood by others. I must remember to explain it. Instead, I find myself staying home. It's just easier.

I've come across a publication from Brain Injury Canada: Returning to Work Following an Acquired Brain Injury

– A self-paced guidebook and resources to help support you along the way. It's written in an easy-to-read format. I read, "Return to work is a process—not an event." That makes sense to me. As I flip through the pages, I randomly read short bits and pieces, "You may also be putting pressure on yourself to return to work as you possibly become impatient with the pace of your recovery. And because your identity may be closely linked with your employment, you may have the sense that if you could just get back to work, you will feel whole or normal again." This resonates with me. It's exactly how I'm feeling. It goes on to say, "It is important to be aware of this. Rushing back to work before you are ready could result in detrimental consequences and could result in a setback to your overall recovery." I need to sit with this; I need to take this in. If I actually stepped away from my computer and stopped pushing to read, would my headaches improve? Would my vision and balance improve? Am I pushing too hard? Would this intentional mental rest allow me to heal enough to get back to work sooner?

## *What I have learned ...*

**Express and receive gratitude.** "When we express gratitude and receive the same, our brain releases dopamine and serotonin, the two crucial neurotransmitters responsible for our emotions, and they make us feel 'good.' They enhance our mood immediately, making us feel happy from the inside." [1]

Remembering to be grateful was a game-changer for me. I didn't make a point of being grateful daily until the end of the first year after my stroke. I wish someone had told me much earlier how very important it is. Expressing gratitude changes your outlook and your perspective.

Consider keeping a daily gratitude journal.

**Use resources.** If you want to explore the possibility of going back to work, this is a great publication: *Return to Work Following an Acquired Brain Injury. A Self-paced Guidebook and Resources to Help Support You Along the Way.* Produced by Brain Injury Canada, it's filled with information such as possible stages of returning to work, reasons for wanting to return to work, establishing a balance, strategies for preparing to leave home (time estimates and planning template), making contact with your employer, pre-return research, workplace policies and employment legislation. There is also a section on learning from others, with personal accounts from people who have gone down this path.

**Stop comparing yourself or your situation to others and their situations.** In particular, I had to stop comparing our financial situation to the circumstances of others in order to find some peace. Once I quit thinking about how much we were lacking and started expressing gratitude for what we had, this turned my attitude around and reduced a ton of stress. Albeit, I didn't come across this revelation until nearly the end of the first year. I'm hoping that, by sharing this with you now, you won't need to wait that long.

"Gratitude makes sense of our past, brings peace for today, and creates a vision for tomorrow." *Melody Beattie, Author*

"Gratitude and attitude are not challenges; they are choices." *Robert Braathe*

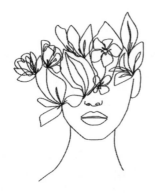

# Month 4

## (August 21- September 20, 2019)

## *August 21–23*

For many years, friends and I have had a Girls' Weekend, usually in the late spring or in the fall. One of our group, my dear friend, has had a year of challenges, so we decide to keep this get-together small, with just three of us rather than the usual five to thirteen women.

We travel to Maple Creek, a small Western Saskatchewan town that has several boutique shops, including a toy store, which is where we begin our shopping day. I'm excited to be here with the girls, to just have some fun. I don't even give a thought to the adverse reactions I've had in the not-so-distant past to being in a store. And then, *wow*, the first store makes my head spin. I try to fight it. I don't want to miss this experience of shopping with my friends—to point out some fun finds and giggle at funny signs on the walls. I feel my balance waver and know I need to immediately step outside before I fall. I find a bistro table out on the street where I sit and enjoy a cold drink while the girls shop. My change in plans works perfectly. It's a beautiful sunny day and I'm quite happy to people-watch in this bustling little prairie town. My friends bring their purchases to me for drop-off and to check on me, and then they carry on. I really don't mind. I'm feeling more accepting of my response to too much visual and audio stimulation. I continue to hope it will be better each time. It helps that my friends know what I've been going through and are encouraging. We've been friends long enough that they know I won't be upset if they carry on with their shopping adventure. We have the rest of the weekend to enjoy one another's company. I know I'll hear their stories and see their purchases when we return to the bed-and-breakfast.

I am so grateful for these forever friends, my cheerleaders in life.

## August 26

A friend is studying Healing Sound Therapy and asked if

I'd be interested in having her practice on me. Treating fellow therapists is something my colleagues and I have done throughout our careers, as it provides such valuable and accurate feedback. I know she values my honesty.

I lie on the massage table as she rings bells—or maybe bowls—throughout the treatment. I have my eyes closed. I feel the need to have my feet on the ground— an odd feeling. I pray fervently that only that which is nourishing and nurturing pass between us. Nourishing and nurturing—it's a prayer that I always pray as a practitioner.

When her hands are on my feet, I experience an unusual numbness all the way up to my ankles, like they've been shot with the same numbing agent my dentist uses. I feel pressure in my head and an odd sensation of scratching on my back, but she isn't touching me there. I'm not sure how long the treatment lasts—thirty minutes, maybe an hour? I know my friend had healing intentions for me. But something about the treatment doesn't feel comfortable. I can't tell what. I appreciate her offer to help. I'm not sure there was noticeable benefit for me. Even though there was no change in my symptoms, I value the opportunity to try different modalities to see what works for me. I often suggested to my massage clients that they may want to try acupuncture, or cranial sacral therapy, or laser treatments when they weren't finding they were benefiting from massage. I think that is the philosophy of most therapists—you always want the best for your clients. Now, I want the best for me and will continue to search out treatments that may help.

## *August 27*

As Blair and I drive to Moose Jaw, my son Jared is on my mind. Today is his 30th birthday. So hard to believe he's that age. *Thank you, Lord, for blessing us with him.* I feel that he—and his sister—have had too much family health drama for their young years. I wish often that this wasn't their reality.

We have an appointment with the facilitator of the Moose Jaw chapter of the Saskatchewan Brain Injury Association. Being here brings back intense memories. Several years ago, Justine and I volunteered as massage therapists at the Saskatchewan ABI (Acquired Brain Injury) Summer Camp in northern Saskatchewan. At the time, I was a registered massage therapist and Justine was a massage therapist in training. The camp had cabins that provided a sort of communal living. Justine and I shared a room with two single beds. The transom window above our door was missing so we could easily hear the conversations of the families in the neighbouring rooms.

Our first day was spent getting to know the medical

histories of many of the campers as we prepared to treat them safely. At the end of that day, after hearing their stories and providing massages, we were emotionally spent. Back in our cabin, lying on our beds, we reached across the narrow space between us and held hands. We needed to share each other's experience and draw on each other's strength. We quietly talked about the amazing progress some of these people had made in working past their injury and adjusting their life to accommodate their new limitations.

At one point, as we lay there holding hands, we heard a woman's voice saying, "What are you doing!? Get your clothes on!" She sounded equally annoyed and exhausted. There were many young people at the camp and I assumed that possibly some attractions were blossoming, and she had come across a young couple. Then we were surprised to hear an older man's voice, her husband's, I assumed, and my perception of the scenario completely changed. My heart went out to the woman. In our short time, this first day of this weekend camp, we had seen many unexpected and what could be deemed inappropriate actions by some of these people who had survived a variety of different brain injuries. She must be exhausted by having to parent her spouse. There was some discussion during the weekend about how marriages are affected by brain injuries. Someone cited a statistic stating that anywhere from 20 to 80 percent of marriages ended in divorce or separation following ten months from the time of injury. I was crushed when I heard that, but I see now how it could be an incredible strain on a marital relationship.

A very friendly fellow seemed to take to Justine and me; he had come for a massage on our first day at the camp. Following that, throughout the weekend he would join us in conversation whenever he'd see us. He would start every sentence with, "Hi, my name is Kevin [not his real name] and I'm forty-one years old" and then he'd carry on with his next thought. We noticed that he was wearing a coat, bright red, even though it was comfortably warm outside.

As we entered the dining hall for supper one night, we heard, "Hi my name is Kevin and I'm forty-one years old. Would it be okay if I joined you ladies for supper?" "Of course," we replied. The volunteers were asked to fill their plates first at the smorg table. Once we returned, Kevin took his turn to go and fill his plate. I noticed that he left his red coat on the chair beside me. I tried desperately to keep an eye on him in the crowd in case he forgot where we were sitting. I didn't want him to lose his coat. I looked away from him for a moment and lost him. I asked Justine to help me look for him. We saw him standing against a wall surveying the crowd, and we watched while he spotted our table and then us. When he reached us, he explained that he leaves his red coat wherever he wants to get back to. He said that his internal GPS was one of the things he'd injured when he hit his head after a slip on some ice. It was an adaptation he'd made to manoeuvre in his new world. I thought, *What a resilient man.* Although this chance meeting happened many years ago, there are times now when I think of him and the memory helps me convince myself that anything's possible. I just need to learn to adjust—to pivot and carry on.

Some of the background stories of the young people at the camp were about car accidents at their grad parties, and even after treatments and therapies, they were unable to work or drive. These stories impacted Justine the most, as she had graduated from high school just a few years earlier. We spoke with the mother of an extremely attractive and well-dressed young man. She said he'd been at the wrong place at the wrong time. He took a shortcut through an alley and for reasons unknown to him, was severely beaten by a group of young men. He was an athlete and a solid student. Now in his early twenties, he had lost all of his forward thinking. He'd tried working at a local A&W but didn't last long. He couldn't process that if something was spilled on the floor it needed to be wiped up to avoid slips and falls. This was just one of the many examples she gave of how his brain injury had affected him. He still enjoys dressing up, she said—it gives him a sense of his old self. He struggles with anger over how his life has changed. I often think of him now. I wish that I understood his frustrations then in the way I do now. I would have loved to talk with him more, maybe just to commiserate, maybe to share a knowing moment of the frustration that is so hard to explain to others.

Those few days at the camp provided one of the best learning experiences of my career as a caregiver. I'm so glad I got to share it with Justine. We both learned so much about compassion, empathy, and resilience. We left the camp with many emotions, including deep respect for the campers and their families. We also recognized the great need for ongoing emotional, financial, and therapeutic support for people with brain injuries.

I also, humbly, felt gratitude for my recovery from the car accident I had in my teens, and that it had not changed my life. In a sad coincidence in our lives, Blair had also been in a car accident in the 1970s, and had suffered severe facial injuries and a head injury. He recovered and came out of it reasonably unscathed. Prior to this camp, we really had no way of knowing just how fortunate we are. My experience at the camp is also the reason I know that there are ABI support groups throughout Saskatchewan. I searched until I found our local chapter. I wish that a referral had been offered to us much earlier and that I didn't need to put so much mental effort into finding the service on my own. But we are connected now, and I will attend monthly meetings. It will be good to talk to others and find out how their recovery has been. I have so many questions.

My remembrance of the ABI Camp makes me acutely aware of how beautifully God has scripted my life. How He brought together our organist and best man at our wedding—their relationship developed quickly and deeply, they married and had a son who would become the smart and compassionate young man who brought me such comfort and confidence in the ambulance. I can still hear his voice accurately and succinctly giving the details of my stroke and status to the stroke team awaiting my arrival in Moose Jaw. This thought of how beautifully I was provided for elicited a feeling of God nudging me with His elbow, *Did you catch that?* I reply, *Yes, I love how you take care of every detail in my book of life.* And then, as I almost feel His arm around my shoulder, *Do you see why you were purposed to help at the ABI Family Camp?* I think, *Yes, thank you for this beautiful foreshadowing. I see the family struggles and am so grateful for my family and friends who are my team. Thank you for Kevin, and the memorable example of how he chose joy and a red coat to help him enjoy his new life. Thank you, Lord, for loving me enough to punctuate my life with these moments that I recognize as God-incidents. Thank you for loving me every moment of my life. For never leaving nor forsaking me.* And then I turn and reverently bow my head as I let Him wrap me in a full, loving embrace.

## *August 29*

Physio appointment today. I go into it remembering what I was told at an earlier appointment—that some people have a rather spontaneous recovery. The physiotherapist referred to it as a light-switch effect; you just wake up one morning with hardly any symptoms. I still wish for that, hope for that, pray for that.

## *September 5*

I have a massage today, and I am less emotionally fragile than I was last time. Venting to my massage therapist and friend feels good as I tell her about how slow my recovery has been. I'm so impatient. I am continuing to struggle with headaches and visual disturbances. She spends more time on my neck and shoulders today. Without speaking of the reason for targeting my neck and shoulders, I know from our training that we hold a lot of tension and emotions in these areas. I'm grateful for her wisdom. I trust that she will treat these areas expertly and with the knowledge that if my emotions begin to intensify, she will back off. I always feel safe in her hands. I know I can tell her what does works for me and what doesn't without offending her, although she has amazing instinct and empathy and always seems to sense when to move on to another area.

## *September 6*

Blair and I are selling Chase the Ace tickets for our local Kinsmen group today. Blair has been volunteering for this service organization for over forty years. We have a quiet spot to sit in the dimly lit pub where the tickets are sold, and enjoy having a coffee and visiting with each other. We're not terribly busy, so it makes for an enjoyable time. The location is close enough to our home that I can walk back when I've had enough. It feels good to have a reason to get out and to be helpful.

## *September 10*

I've been meeting with my family physician every month for him to check on my progress and to keep up with the insurance forms. He feels that I'm still not ready to return to work. Every time I see him we have forms to complete, it seems. I truly appreciate his help.

There's something to be said for living in a small town and going to the same doctor for thirty years, and to know him like we do. I feel reassured in sharing my experiences and frustrations with a professional who knows me from before the stroke. He knows about Blair's health concerns and he understands that my recovery is more than just about getting back to work; it's about getting back to my life, with all its realities and responsibilities. I'm grateful to him.

## September 17–19

A dear friend and I are on a three-day trip to Winnipeg, on an organized bus trip. I am really happy about spending time with her. We stay at a hotel with a casino—we have both enjoyed a little "play time" in the past. Not sure how that will go now, with the cacophony and busyness of a casino. The bus trip also includes shopping. I've brought some stitching in case my head doesn't allow me to spend time in front of a slot machine, or in a store.

Initially, I enjoy the mindless time and have been lucky enough to be playing off of the casino's money. But I've been here an hour and I know it's been too long. I find my friend to tell her I'm going to go back to the room. She's very understanding. She's going to stay and play some more. I'm glad she's comfortable doing that. I don't want her to feel that she needs to watch over me, or worse, entertain me.

Well, let's just say I get a lot of stitching done during this trip. That's okay. I'm excited to do some of the girlfriend things we've done in the past. I'm still forgetting that I have challenges until I try to do what I've always done before—play at the casino, go into a store, stay up late to catch up with an old friend. This is very different from our past trips. We've been friends for over forty years and have supported each other through so much—the loss of her parents and then her son, and the loss of my sister. She provided my home away from home when I was taking courses in the city near her. We've always enjoyed travelling and being together. When we were young and single, we'd go to parties and if it were a dull party, we'd turn to each other and one would say, "What is this?" and in unison we would say, "A good time!" and then laugh. Through the ups and downs of life, this dear friend has stayed by my side. She makes my life "a good time!"

## *What I have learned ...*

**CPP Disability.** I include this information about CPP Disability insurance here only because there is usually a four-month waiting period to consider. This is just information to keep in your back pocket until you know it's time to take action. Regardless of what the government website says, pretty much everyone I've spoken with about this has said that from the time they applied to being approved took six to seven months rather than the four-month period suggested on the website. You'll want to keep that in mind if you know that your disability insurance will run out after a year. It's so hard to know at this point if you'll be back to work in six or seven months or if you'll have long-lasting impairments. The link for more information is: *https://www.canada.ca/en/services/ benefits/publicpensions/cpp/cpp-disability-benefit/apply.html*

The instructions on that website are:

You should apply as soon as you develop a mental or physical condition that:

- prevents you from working regularly at any job
- is long-term and of unknown duration, or is likely to result in death

Do not delay in sending your completed application form.

**Accept vulnerability.** I'd explain my fourth month as a period of a little less frustration and maybe a little more vulnerability. I came across this quote from Brené Brown and felt encouraged by it. I hope it encourages you: "Vulnerability is not winning or losing. It's having the courage to show up when you can't control the outcome."

I wish for you the courage it takes to keep showing up. You have what it takes to make your life worth living.

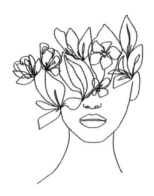

# Month 5
## (September 21–October 20, 2019)

## *September 23*

It's been four months since my stroke. Because I have no visible physical impairments I continue to question if I'm really disabled. Surely my brain will heal and I won't always be like this. Or will I? I don't know—my daily accomplishments are still so far from what I used to be able to do.

A few weeks ago, I remembered that I had critical illness insurance. *Do I qualify?* I wondered. *Is my condition "bad enough" to warrant it?* Some days it sure is, but I'm still hoping I'll get past this, like I did after the car accident in 1975. I decide to submit a claim and let the insurer decide. I am seeing my family doctor today to begin the process of filling out the forms.

## September 24

I have returned to yin yoga classes. This is one of my favourite self-care times. I enjoy the dark, quiet space—the focus on nothing more than my breath, the opportunity to move my body in different twists, turns, and stretches that I wouldn't otherwise do, and the soothing voice of our yoga instructor as she encourages us to hold the pose for periods of three to five minutes. I didn't realize how much I'd been shallow-breathing. Deep breathing while doing yoga feels like I'm making short, quick gasps, as if I'm going to cry. I was unaware of how much I needed this. The final, restorative, resting pose comes too quickly. I leave, looking forward to classes for the next eight weeks.

## October 3

A new staff member has been hired at work to cover my desk. I'm not sure how long she's been there. She has called me a few times for questions as she gets her bearings. I've even popped in a few times to help her out.

My physical office location has moved to accommodate the addition of new staff and my files are now in boxes. This adds to my feeling of disorientation. I can't imagine how extra stressful this is for the new employee. Today I will be training her on the database I created specifically for my job. I learned the software and then created a database to make searching for statistical data easier. The trick is to be able to wrap my post-stroke head around how to access these tools again.

We start our session with her questions—how to deal with certain donation requests; where to find stats; how to address the budget. They're important questions. Some I can answer and some I can't find the answers for in my memory bank. All the questions are draining my brain battery. *Hang in there,* I encourage myself.

It feels very odd having someone settling into my "domain." I have an internal battle going on—I want to encourage and help her as much as I can, while still grappling with the desire to not let go of my work world.

I'm not sure how helpful I am but I assure her that she can call me with questions. As I walk home, I have the sense that it's over. In my gut I know that I am really lacking the cognitive abilities needed to carry on my job to the professional level I had achieved in the past. I have very mixed emotions—I'm so glad my member relation responsibilities and our customers' needs are being met, but a part of me feels like I've been replaced. Permanently.

## October 4

My mom was born in Saskatchewan and moved to Ontario as a preschooler. She is a very accomplished woman. As well as giving birth to five of us in just six years, she is a talented artist, and was a successful restauranteur, entrepreneur (ceramics and antiques), and volunteer (4H leader). Mom moved from Ontario to Saskatchewan in 2006 and took up residence at The Lodge in Rockglen, which provided comfortable senior housing that included activities such as music, cards, jigsaw puzzles and daily coffee visits—all the things she enjoyed.

She often said she remembered the Saskatchewan winds and how they made her head and body hurt so was hesitant to move back—but I was glad when she did. It has been good to have mom here as our children were growing up. In 2010, she moved from Rockglen to Assiniboia and eight years later, she moved to a private care home.

This April, Mom flew back to Ontario to explore senior housing options there. Unfortunately, the waiting lists are well over a year long and without suitable housing, it looks like Mom is going to be returning to Saskatchewan.

My initial reaction is, *I'm not okay. I'm not better. I can't take care of myself, let alone care for Mom. And this is too much to add to Blair's plate right now. He is doing all the driving for both of us. Is it too much for him if we add driving Mom to her appointments as well?* She had a pacemaker inserted in August and would need follow-up care. *Lord, please give us the strength to do this. Please give me wisdom to know when to say "no" and when to be the caregiving daughter who needs to step up to the plate. Please Lord, keep Blair in your loving arms. Please don't let this extra stress and responsibility wear him down to the point that he's not able to keep fighting the cancer. Please allow my healing to continue. Please guide me to keep Mom safe and cared for. In Jesus' mighty name I pray.*

Luckily, I was able to find an apartment for Mom within a block of our home so I will be able to easily check in on her. Thanks to our caring community members, I have had several responses to requests for affordable furnishings. Mom wants to try an apartment and be independent. I think that she needs to be in a care home, but I am willing to help her give the apartment a try.

## *October 6*

Mom has arrived and I'm proud of how cute and homey I have made the apartment. But I'm exhausted and not in a great mood. I want to be more welcoming but I am already feeling too overwhelmed. With all the strength and courage I can muster, I acknowledge to myself that Mom has moved back to my care today. I will do this and do it well. With all my heart I know it's the right move for Mom.

I am sensing that my healing progress has stopped. I've returned to increased anxiety, increased visual disturbances, decreased sleep, and increased memory loss. Simple tasks like hooking up TV and power for Mom have been monumental. I have tasked myself to do only one of these items per day and some days even that is too much. *Lord, we need you more than ever now. Thank you for the support of our families and community.*

## October 8

I started today with physio and then, after a brief rest at home, I went to a meeting with the local chapter of the Acquired Brain Injury (ABI) support group. The participants have survived a variety of life incidents, including brain cancer and strokes. Today our general discussion is about sleep. My question is, "Does anyone else get a headache as soon as they lie down for the night, or shortly afterward?" Yes. Several do. I'm not alone! Someone *gets* me and what I'm going through. I could cry. I didn't realize how alone I've been feeling until just now. I receive valuable advice today—when I'm ready for bed, I will try getting the first part of the evening's sleep while reclined in a chair, and then move to the bed for the rest of the night.

This group gets me! Voicing my concerns before felt like complaining and sometimes came out as excuses because I didn't want to participate in certain activities, anticipating that it would exacerbate my evening headaches. It is easier to avoid groups of more than four and group conversations than to explain how tiring taking in information, processing and coming up with an intelligent response is. Explaining this to family and friends feels like I am making excuses not to go out. Taking part in shopping or shows makes my head spin. Does this sound like another excuse to stay home? All of this results in nighttime headaches that are both concerning and painful. Does everyone with brain injuries hurt like this? It is easier staying home and staying comfortable, but I am also feeling left behind. I trust my friends will still be there for me when this gets easier.

One more appointment for the day. I meet with a Home Care supervisor at Mom's apartment to set up her home care visits and Meals on Wheels. We agree to home care visits twice a week, and they will stay while Mom has her shower so she can feel safe doing that by herself. We book meals to be delivered five days a week. This already feels like some weight has been taken off my shoulders.

To help Mom with this new routine, we put everything on a large desk calendar for her, as well as on a calendar on her fridge. My mother's home care team has left a binder on top of her fridge where they will record notes. There is also a space for me to add comments or concerns. I feel very supported and much more confident in Mom's and my ability to do this!

## October 9

Last night, I tried the recommended bedtime routine suggested at the ABI meeting. We have a recliner right in our couch so I lay back, put a pillow beside my head to roll up against, and I had the best sleep I've had in months. I woke after about an hour and then went off to bed. No headache all night. Brilliant! I am so grateful for this wonderful night's sleep.

## October 15

The yin yoga classes have been amazing. Some days I feel like it's the only time I can safely deeply inhale and exhale. I feel such a difference in my breathing from the start of the class to the end, seventy-five minutes later.

## *October 18*

Mom has been back in Assiniboia for ten days. I've gone over at least once a day to help reset her remote or find her keys or something else she'd misplaced. Just as I had expected, she is more confused after the move.

But I am startled today by a phone call from home care. The volunteers had gone twice to her suite to drop off her day's meal. There was no answer either time. Immediately I wonder if she had fallen in her suite, so I dash right over to check on her. No Mom. I check her calendar to see if she had written anything that would explain where she was. The first thing I notice is a Post-it note with my handwriting. It's for an appointment in a few days in Regina. I don't remember that appointment and it's not in my calendar. Is this a note that may have fallen out of her address book, an old note from when she lived here in Assiniboia previously? I make some phone calls but do not find out what this appointment was for. Is my memory slipping more than I thought?

I can see her calendar had been written on, scribbled out, and the same notations written back in. Mom is always so neat and organized with her calendars. Just looking at the mess of the month's notations makes me feel anxious for her. She often voices her concerns about being confused and forgetful. I am sad to see such a visual display of her failing abilities. I feel her distress as I look at it. This isn't going well for her. Why didn't she say something to me? I know she wants to be independent. I must find her and find out what's going on for her.

Blair is away with the car. I am on foot. I walk around her building, then head downtown to the local seniors' centre. I can feel my brain battery draining from the emotional stress and worry. I go into an alley and cry for a short time. I just need a moment to reset, to pray, to self-soothe with some deep breaths.

A woman sees me and stops to check on me. I tell her that I can't find my mom. The woman happens to be on her way to the seniors' centre so I ask her to keep an eye out for my mother. She assures me that our community is small enough that we'll find her. I appreciate her caring comments. I've composed myself enough to carry on.

I think that maybe Mom has decided to treat herself to Chinese food, which was one of her favourite restaurant meals here in town. I head there, and, sure enough, she is there with a friend. I want to not be angry, to not scold her as if she were a child. I think about her calendar and how unsettling this move must be for her. I want to be happy for her that she has reconnected with an old friend over lunch. I get my emotions in check enough to tell her I'm happy that she's out for some Chinese food. I also tell her it's important that if she's not going to be home for her meal deliveries that she needs to let me know.

I stop over to see her later in the day. I want to know how she thinks she's coping. Is she feeling comfortable and safe being on her own? I'm still concerned about the state of her calendar. She said she feels like she's being smothered by having to be home for the meals and with those people checking in on her all the time. We agree to cut back the home care visits to once a week and the meals back to three times a week.

It's been an unsettling day. I'm glad Mom has enjoyed her outing and that we have a new plan in place. My anxiety is elevated a notch with the reduction of home care check-ins. I'm going to do my best to work within Mom's comfort. I'm hoping she'll manage better as she finds her new routine. For today, I can only trust that both Mom and I are adjusting and that this will get easier.

## *What I have learned ...*

### Sleep is vital to your recovery.

According to the neurorehabilitation specialist Henry Hoffman, "Quality sleep has many benefits, especially for stroke survivors. Getting a good night's sleep supports neuroplasticity, the brain's ability to restructure and create new neural connections in healthy parts of the brain, allowing stroke survivors to re-learn movements and functions."

### From Hoffman's writings, I learned some tips to improve sleep:

*Try to stay consistent in your sleep times* – Try to go to bed and wake at the same time each day. A healthy length of sleep is eight hours, so let that be your target.

*Avoid daytime naps* – I try to avoid naps, but some days it feels like it's not my choice. However, when I don't nap during the day I certainly sleep better at night.

*Watch what you eat and drink before bedtime* - Avoid overeating before bedtime. In fact, any eating two hours before you go to bed for the night isn't recommended. Caffeine, alcohol, and nicotine are also discouraged late in the day.

*Create a calm environment* – A room that is cool, quiet, and dark is best. Did you know that research shows that clutter in your space affects anxiety levels, sleep, and the ability to focus? This is a good argument for keeping your bedroom tidy. Video screens really stimulate your brain, so you want to set them aside. If you're not able to read, this would be a good time to listen to an audio book or a sleep meditation until you're ready to sleep.

*Address your worries* – This might be as simple as having a note pad beside your bed to write down what's on your mind. Once written, set it aside with the intention of dealing with it the next day. I find that deep breathing or any type of meditation is also a good way to settle my mind for the night.

*Stay active* – Activity is wonderful for encouraging sleep, especially if you can be active outside. (But give yourself a few hours before bedtime as a window to minimize any overly stimulating activities.)

This is a time to draw on our courage and hope. Once we're able to rest, we gain renewed strength and clarity to move on.

> "Perhaps strength doesn't reside in having never been broken but in the courage required to grow strong in the broken places." – *Necole Stephens*

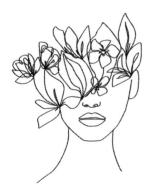

# Month 6
## (October 21–November 20, 2019)

## *October 22*

What a great day! I wake up feeling refreshed. My balance feels better, my thoughts clearer, my attitude more positive, even the sun seems like it's shining brighter. I recall my first visit with my physiotherapist, when she told me that for some people there is a "light-switch" day—they wake up and feel that life is pretty much as it was before the stroke. *Is this that day?*

I will remember this day as the best I've had since I had my stroke, and it will be my benchmark day—I will compare every day with how great this day feels. (For months, I did compare my good days with "my October

22 day," but it would be more than a year before I felt this good again.)

I attend a yin yoga class. These classes are so helpful for my anxiety and just to help me consciously deep-breathe.

## October 24

Mom has asked for another calendar because her calendar is missing the month of October. I realize that she had thrown away the page and written her October appointments on the November page. The dates aren't lining up which added to her confusion. I told her I'd print fresh October and November pages. They won't match the rest of her calendar, but they will be cleaner and easier to read.

## October 25

My headaches are getting worse. I feel so frustrated because I can't identify what is setting them off nor can I identify what is making them worse. I'm sure they are connected to me spending more time on my computer and possibly worrying about Mom. Since I can't seem to stay away from screen time, I have decided to pack up my computer today and leave it in the box until my headaches subside. I am hoping that won't be for long, but I feel like I need to let my brain heal and not hurt.

## *October 28*

I manage to get my critical illness forms completed and faxed in to the insurance company. All I can do now is hope.

I see my optometrist, who puts a temporary prism on my glasses to see if it will help with my feeling of unsteadiness. Ideally the prism will help my brain transition more easily between my near-sighted left eye and far-sighted right eye. So far, having the prism on my glasses makes me feel the same as when I first began to wear my trifocals years ago—like my balance is off and the walls are closing in on me. With my trifocals, it took a week before I could see without being aware of the transition lines in the lenses. I sure hope this helps—at least enough that I'm more confident to walk a distance alone.

I arrive home to an email from the critical illness insurance company informing me that they will not be granting me any benefits because a transient ischemic attack does not meet the criteria for a stroke. A stroke, they explain, is an acute cerebrovascular event with onset of new neurological symptoms and deficits that last for more than thirty days, and does not include transient ischemic attacks. The email states that a doctor on their Medical Board reviewed my file and agreed with the decision.

I am shocked and dismayed to read this, because I know I did not have a transient ischemic attack (TIA)! It seems that my surgeon inadvertently identified my stroke as a TIA, which by definition has residual effects resolving within twenty-four hours. That obviously isn't true in my case. The surgeon had already identified it to me and in other reports as a stroke. I'll have to call the insurance office tomorrow and clarify that this was an unfortunate mistake.

## *October 29*

At the recommendation of my physiotherapist, today I am seeing a physiotherapist in Regina who specializes in vestibular conditions. The vestibular system includes the parts of the inner ear and brain that process the sensory information involved with controlling balance and eye movements. If disease or injury damages these processing areas, vestibular disorders can result.

The physiotherapist runs a series of tests, such as tracking my eye movement and my ability to balance on one foot. I tell the physiotherapist during my session that even conversations seem to be tiring for me. She explains to me that the brain is like an hourglass sand timer—information comes into the top, and the narrow part is the processing centre. When the processing centre gets overwhelmed, it has to shut down to "reset," making output (speaking) difficult at that time. This explanation makes complete sense to me. When my sudden fatigue comes on I get very quiet; it's just too much effort to talk. I don't feel like I have a choice; I simply need to sleep when this happens.

The tests are very tiring for me and I lie down to rest as the physiotherapist writes her notes.

The "Impression of condition on initial assessment" from this physiotherapist is: "*This 61-year-old female presented following CVA* [cardiovascular accident, also known as a stroke] *in May of 2019 with vestibular dysfunction, motion sensitivity and disequilibrium* [a general feeling of being off balance or being unable to remain upright and move through space with confidence. Most commonly, this occurs during standing and walking]. *This presents primarily to be affecting the central vestibular system with increased reliance on her visual system rather than her vestibular and somatosensory* [relating to or denoting a sensation such as pressure, pain, or warmth which can occur anywhere in the body in contrast to one localized at a sense organ such as sight, balance, or taste] *input systems. She also displays high level of fatigue with increased stimulation through these areas.*"

In other words, my internal system that makes me adjust and feel 'balanced' was impaired by the stroke. She found that rather than the system automatically making adjustments to keep my eyes level with the horizon, I was relying on making conscious adjustments to what I am looking at. Furthermore, she noted my high level of fatigue as I tried to anticipate and compensate for this loss of balance.

The physiotherapist wants to share with me exercises that should help my condition. Between my fatigue and having just received my prism for my glasses yesterday, the idea of thinking about exercises is too much for my overloaded brain and we book a return appointment.

I sleep during the drive home.

## *November 1*

This morning, I email my reply to the caseworker at the critical illness company, explaining that the surgeon must have erroneously recorded a TIA. I ask her to review the reports from my family physician and the ER doctor that clearly identify my episode as a stroke. The caseworker replied, asking for the surgeon to confirm that his diagnosis as TIA was incorrect. My report summary said the diagnosis was stroke, but somewhere in the body of the surgeon's report he wrote "TIA." I am embarrassed to have to call the doctors and ask them to reach out to the critical illness company on my behalf.

I share this problem with my family physician, and he writes to the company on November 3 to confirm I'd had a stroke. This, however, wasn't good enough for them, so I have to contact the surgeon. He was less than impressed with the insurance company and said that it was obviously an incorrect statement because a TIA doesn't last more than twenty-four hours—but he was gracious enough to send them an amendment to his report.

I feel so discouraged because this is all so hard on my head. I am frustrated and emotional about the uncertainty of this situation and the time it is costing my medical professionals.

From 1986-1987, I used my training as a Fellow of the Life Management Institute (FLMI) to secure a job with Co-operators Life Insurance in Regina as a head office life underwriter. My job included reviewing life insurance applications to assess if the applicant had a significant risk that could possibly create a claim prematurely. We knew what questions to ask to clarify whether or not the applicant was insurable at a standard rate, rated for increased premium, or declined. Having been an insurance underwriter for two years, I knew the process and therefore knew that the file review had been handled poorly.

## November 5

Blair drives me to another Acquired Brain Injury (ABI) group meeting, in Assiniboia. Today the group discusses some brain games that will safely stimulate our brains. We are told about some free apps for use on a computer or phone. Unfortunately, looking at a screen still creates headaches for me, so I don't even keep the list.

Later, I go to a yin yoga class, and then on to a presentation by a motivational speaker. I am so ready to be feeling better about my life. The presentation was so good! It had been organized by the Assiniboia Mental Health and Wellness Team, and was extremely well attended, including people from neighbouring farming communities who were struggling with recent droughts and financial stresses.

This has been a very busy day and my head is really hurting, but I'm so glad I went to the presentation. I am feeling far more positive.

## November 7

I am with the physiotherapist in Regina to learn vestibular exercises. Several are eye exercises, including one that requires me to move my eyes around a large clock made of Post-it notes placed on the wall. Interestingly, she tells me not to do this exercise for more than two minutes at a time, and to follow it with at least ninety minutes of rest. She explained that brain stress is cumulative and, in her experience, extending the exercise too long can actually cause hallucinations if there is not sufficient time to rest. I'm glad she mentioned that, because I am definitely an over-achiever and would have done this exercise for much longer than I should have, thinking more was better.

Today I also have an appointment to take the prism off my glasses to see if it has made any difference in my balance. I will try going without it for a week or so. The prism is temporary and can be reapplied to my glasses if needed. Did it help? I'm not sure if it was just good to no longer have the lines in my vision or if my balance had somewhat improved.

## November 10

I am feeling very introspective today. I am thinking, *What if...God gave me struggles to prepare me to be of service to other people? I have experienced so much...*

- a major car accident in Grade 12
- the loss of a sister to breast cancer
- a husband with stage IV cancer
- financial struggles
- a stroke that took away the busy life I'd known.

All of this is not without blessings…

- my life was spared in the car accident, and after a year of healing I had a new-found affinity for learning that took me down several exciting and interesting career paths
- my sister's battle with cancer prepared us for Blair's
- Blair has outlived his doctors' prognoses by several years
- financial struggles keep us grateful for all the blessings we've had. Our family has never missed a meal, been homeless, or been more than a few weeks without an opportunity for income
- I have more time for Blair
- slowing down helps me to search inward and reflect.

Having considered all of this, my prayer is: *God use me, make me Your instrument, open the eyes of my heart so I can see Your purpose for me, fill me with the excitement and energy of knowing that I am on Your path and fulfilling Your purpose for my time on this earth.*

It feels good to have this time of reflection. Since my stroke almost six months ago, I know I have experienced cognitive impairments. I long for that feeling of wanting to do something, to feel the spark (God's spark) that leads me. I feel like I want to—and need to—keep writing.

## *November 11*

I am continuing to look inward.

What if: The stroke was a precious lesson? For seven hours I couldn't speak. Was this meant to help me have a new respect for the privilege and power of speech? Are my words encouraging, thoughtful, uplifting, kind, respectful?

*Lord, please guide my every word and keep it pleasing to You.*

What if losing my ability to comprehend written word was meant to help me appreciate all the training I've had the opportunity to receive in the past? Maybe, safely stored in my grey matter, I already have all the information I need to serve others.

What if my stroke was an answer to my prayers in a way I hadn't planned? On my 2019 vision board (something I have created for the past five years), I had posted words including: *Freedom - Pay off our vehicle - Get more shuteye - Take a break! - Give thanks! - Get healthy and fit – Relax.* All of these have already happened. What I hadn't put on my vision board but pray for often is to have more time with Blair. I have really enjoyed this time with Blair, our daily caring for each other—sharing the responsibility of caregiver for each other in a way that makes our bond even stronger. Am I overthinking this? Maybe, but *What if?*

## November 13

Blair has driven Mom and me to Regina for her pacemaker check. She seems quiet and anxious and is tearing up easily. I ask her if living in the apartment is too much. She admits that it is and says that moving back to the care home might be a better idea, but worries that it's too much work for me to arrange after I had just made all the arrangements for her apartment and furnishings. I assure her that most of the furniture was on loan until we knew if she'd be able to stay on her own. She seems relieved to hear that. I explain that it won't be too hard to disconnect utilities and give her notice to let the apartment go. I assure her that we will figure the rest out as we go. I can't imagine how tough this is for her. I trust that she knows how very much we care for her and that all we want is for her to be safe.

She's been back long enough now to know how much I'm struggling with my healing. This only seems to add to her guilt. I assure her that if we can get her a bed at the care home, we'll get back to her old routine and we'll all settle in and be fine. We hold each other in a long embrace.

A dear friend had told me about a reflexologist she

went to for an "emotional reflexology" treatment. This made sense to me. In my massage training I studied— and in my practice, I experienced—how an emotional trauma can leave a physical reaction in a person's body. While massaging I'd often have clients experience SomatoEmotional releases (SER)—the release of emotional energy that was being held in the body. If emotion cannot be expressed or released at the time it was generated, or if a trauma is accompanied by one or more strong emotions, the particular emotions may become trapped in tissues of the body. SomatoEmotional Release is the process of discovering and releasing or redirecting the emotion or emotional energy.

I decide to see this reflexologist. Even though I had an understanding of the treatment, I do what I always do—I enter the appointment with prayers for protection and healing. I stay awake for probably only ten minutes of the treatment.

Before I fell asleep, she finds spots on my foot identifying an area of concern and says, "Something happened in 1975 that shook your confidence for most of the rest of your life." At first, I thought, *Seriously?*

Then, I recalled my injuries from my car accident in 1975. With my left leg in a cast, I wasn't able to board the school bus, so I rode to school daily with the teacher.

My brain fog was intense for nearly a year and learning was difficult—I eventually needed a tutor. Also, I lost my front tooth and that added to my lack of confidence.

After identifying those issues, she works on the spot while having me speak positive affirmations...I am worthy, I am strong, I am confident, I am smart, and so on. As the tenderness at the pressure point subsides, I really feel much better.

Even though I am in a light sleep through most of this appointment, I can hear her speaking positive affirmations as she works on my feet.

At the end, I feel amazing! Like a weight has been lifted. My anxiety, the internal jittery feeling I have had for years, is gone.

She suggests that I use sleep meditations to help with sleep and to continue with positive affirmations.

## November 14

In this time of healing and reflecting, I continue to be highly introspective and speculative—frequently asking myself those "what if?" questions. Today's was: What if the stroke's occurrence on the date of our 31st wedding anniversary wasn't happenstance but a God-incident? Was He showing me that Blair and I will now have more time to spend with each other? So, is it by accident that my stroke happened on our wedding anniversary? I have to believe it was part of God's perfect plan.

Without a doubt, Blair and the kids have stepped up and taken amazing care of me, and they always have. My heart is filled to overflowing. What if I needed to see that—more than I knew—God has provided the opportunity? God is good.

## *November 15*

Good news—there is a bed available for Mom on November 25 at the care home where she lived before she moved back to Ontario. They were able to offer her a room just down the hall from her old room, so she knows who her neighbours will be. We go to look at her new room and sign the papers. She is welcomed back with open arms.

I just need to push through the next ten days of selling or returning the furniture we acquired last month. Arrange disconnects and reconnects. Prepare for the physical move of her bed, dresser, table, and chairs. Do the final cleaning.

## *November 19*

I am excited to receive a call from the critical illness insurance company. I had first submitted the application on October 28. I'm expecting a decision in my favour as I'd duly contacted all the doctors they sought more information from to clarify that I'd had a stroke and not a TIA. Nope! Now they want me to prove that I have cognitive impairment beyond thirty days as stated in the policy. (As I described in Chapter 2, on the day that I was to have a cognitive assessment by the occupational therapist, I was too tired after completing the mini mental-status test, so we said we'd do the cognitive assessment another day. That never happened.)

The caseworker on my file said that I would now have to complete a professional Neuropsychological Assessment, at my own expense. She also said she would keep my file open only until January 23, 2020. If this testing is not completed by then, my file will be closed. What does this mean? What is this test? I need to find out.

## *November 20*

My Netflix account was hacked three days ago, and today I see that my Facebook has been hacked. This is too much!! I find it so hard to work through this. My head hurts. I need to change passwords, and I can't remember how! Calm down. One thing at a time. Start with bank accounts. Do other changes another day. *Lord, please protect my data until I can make changes to protect it.*

Determined to make self-care a high priority, I have booked a massage for today. Each time I go, I feel less like crying and more able to enjoy moments of relaxation.

## *What I have learned ...*

**Reach out for help.** This was a hard lesson to learn. I've always been a take-charge kinda gal, so reaching out doesn't come easy for me. I'm so relieved for the help when I do finally reach out. I was so grateful for the support of Home Care Services for Mom, the Acquired Brain Injury support group, and the physiotherapists who provide such helpful information. Although we can easily get caught up in our own world of recovery, it's important to not get so focused on our own suffering and worry that we are unable to see there are times we need to ask for help.

I feel like reaching out is a sign of weakness, but I have learned that it truly is an act of courage and strength. Be open to blessing those around you with the opportunity to make your life a little easier.

**Consider sleep meditation.** There is a lot of science behind how meditation can help lay down new brain pathways. In their book, **Meditations to Change Your Brain,** Rick Hanson, PhD and Richard Mendius, MD report how meditation can help reduce cortisol, the hormone associated with stress. In the studies, meditation increased the natural melatonin levels to help with more restful sleep. It can also encourage greater focus, emotional control, and thoughtful decision making.

The sleep meditations I listened to are Dauchsy Sleep Meditations. I have to say I was a little distrusting at first; I was naively afraid that maybe someone talking to me in my sleep could put the suggestion in my head that robbing a bank was okay, or something similarly bizarre. What I found, after listening, was that I had markedly increased quality and quantity of sleep. The topics are varied in the Dauchsy series; for example, they cover gratitude, healing, creativity, love attraction, and prosperity. (I definitely feel that I have greater peace of mind and feel more optimistic during the day after having listened to a sleep meditation. I find that the sleep meditations lasting no longer than two hours are the best for me, for some reason. Longer ones seem to always wake me at some point, and then I have a hard time getting back to sleep. I continue to listen to sleep meditations three to four nights a week).

"Be strong enough to stand alone, smart
enough to know when you need help, and brave
enough to ask for it." *Author unknown*

"Don't be shy about asking for help. It doesn't mean
you're weak, it only means you're wise."
*Author unknown*

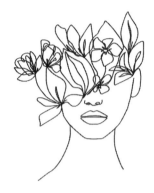

# Month 7
## (November 21–December 20, 2019)

### *November 21*

It's been exactly six months since my stroke. Today is the
follow-up carotid ultrasound to see how my left carotid
artery has recovered from the surgery. I will receive the
results in about a week.

### *November 22*

I do some research into neuropsychological assessment
and find that there are two psychologists in Saskatchewan
who do this formal test. I need the test to prove to
the critical insurance company that I have cognitive

impairment beyond thirty days. I email the psychologist in Regina for further details. The test is lengthy and requires two days in the city. It would be about seventeen billable hours at $210 per hour. I could cry. There is no way I will take over three thousand dollars from our already tight finances in the hope that my insurance application will be approved. I am very concerned that we would go through this testing and then find that the insurance company has another hoop for us to jump through. I thanked the psychologist for her quick response, told her that our finances were tight because of both our health conditions, and explained that unless there is a benevolent fund we could apply to for help in covering the fee, we will have to pass.

## *November 25*

I'm happy today to be moving Mom back into the care home. It's good for her to see familiar faces and get back into a familiar routine. I'm incredibly relieved to know that she is being cared for. I feel like I can now return my focus to my healing. Prior to my stroke, paying her bills and driving her to appointments were effortless. Since my stroke, being able to figure out online bill payments is very challenging, if I can figure them out at all. I'm still not driving, so taking Mom to appointments lies on Blair's shoulders. Thankfully, he's able to drive and is very gracious about driving us to Regina on days when I'm sure he'd rather rest. It's not easy, but we're managing. Mom is so grateful to have our help. I love her to bits.

As today winds down, I can already feel the physical relief of sharing Mom's care with the staff of the care home. My shoulders no longer feel like they're hovering around my ears; I feel looser, and my breath is slower and more relaxed. I can feel myself exhaling. And sleep, precious refreshing sleep, envelops me.

## *November 26*

It's Sunday, and I've just received the most unbelievable email from the psychologist in Regina. She has had a cancellation for December 9–10 and says she would waive much of her fee and do the assessment for $1200 if I'd like to take this newly available appointment. What a relief! It feels like someone is really on our side and is trying to help us out! We had already checked with our group insurance companies and they would cover $800 toward this assessment. I absolutely will take this appointment. *Thank you, Lord!*

## *November 28*

I receive the results of the follow-up carotid ultrasound, and it showed that there was greater than 50 percent stenosis both on my left and right side. That seems to me like quite a blockage following a surgery that was meant to clean out my carotid artery. I ask the surgeon if he is concerned. He explains that because I had a "flap" over the area where the carotid was opened up, the flap may have just had a wrinkle in it when they did the ultrasound. I ask how I would know if it was already starting to develop additional plaque. He said I'd have symptoms, and we could talk about it then. Have symptoms? Like, another stroke? Our discussion doesn't ease my concerns, nor does it make me more confident that the worst is behind me.

## *December 1*

Maybe because I'm sleeping better—maybe because Mom is settling so well at the care home—maybe because I know my work responsibilities at the Co-op are being handled—maybe because of the peace and deep breathing my yoga practice has restored—I'm feeling stronger. I'm pretty tired of feeling like I'm always in fight or flight mode. I'm not loving the person I am right now—I feel like I'm always angry about one thing or another. So I'm putting my foot down. *Today it's time to recreate me! I can still do lots of things, so I will focus on that and work with my strengths.* It feels good and positive to make this proclamation.

## *December 2*

I have been hearing that Indian Head Massage (based on traditional Ayurvedic healing in India) is helpful in relieving headaches and improving sleep. A local therapist has recently taken the training and has asked if I'd like to come in for a treatment and provide some feedback. As with most types of massage, I fall asleep. My head feels good afterward, but maybe it's simply because of the sleep. I feel a little groggier than I do after a usual massage treatment. I'll try this again. As I've told my massage clients over the years, "It's okay to try different treatments to find out what works best for you." I'm taking my own advice!

## *December 9–10*

At 9 a.m., I begin my neuropsychological assessment, with no idea what to expect. I still have days when I question whether my limitations are really that bad. Am I just not trying hard enough? I'm apprehensive and yet curious to know how much impairment there is. The test starts with some fun and simple games—rebuilding blocks into shapes as they appear on a diagram. This is an enjoyable mental challenge at first. But when it becomes more challenging, I have a flashback to the day of my stroke, in that dark room where I felt I had no information, no thoughts, no idea how to proceed. Oh, this scares me. I cry uncontrollably. I am so embarrassed. I gladly take the offer of a break. I have a similar reaction when the next test of repeating visual information gets difficult, so we take another break. I'm so tired. After a lunch break, the testing continues until 4 p.m. I am so glad to be done for today. But I am smiling.

I am staying with a friend, and I decide to take a bus to her place rather than bother her for a ride. I have a quick nap on the bus and become disoriented. Then I find that the bus doesn't run all the way to my friend's house at this hour, so I have to walk the rest of the way, a kilometre or more. Fortunately, I'm dressed fairly warmly. I make it to a church about a half-kilometre from her house and stop there to call her. It's -25C and just too cold to walk any further. Even with the nap on the bus, I feel mentally fatigued from the testing. I am so glad that the church doors are open and a group of women are about to have a meeting. My cell battery has died, so I ask one of the women if she has a charging cable so I can charge my phone enough to make the call for a ride. In a short time, my friend answers the phone and chuckles—she is on her way to this very church to join this meeting!

My friend drops me off and returns to her meeting at the church. I enter the house and check if anyone is home. The house is quiet and I am relieved that I don't have to involve myself in conversation or a review of the happenings of the day. I crawl under the big, beautiful duvet and just sleep.

Day two of the assessment is less of a mental test and more of a test of verbal responses to questions. For part of this day, I'm asked to have a long-time friend join us to give another account of my life before and after my stroke. As this friend, a former college schoolmate, shares some of her perspective, I feel sad that I'm not the person I used to be for her. Not as upbeat, energetic, and fun-loving. (She is careful with her words to not be hurtful but wants the psychologist to understand the changes she has observed.) She says she has seen me cry more since the stroke than she'd seen me cry in the forty years we'd known each other.

The last of the testing involves questions on a computer. I explain that looking at the screen creates headaches but I'd work quickly and try to finish. And I did it!

At the end of the two days of testing, I feel some embarrassment over how quickly I became overwhelmed by parts of the tests. On the other hand, some tests made me feel more confident that I hadn't lost everything, as I could respond quite intelligently to some questions and challenges. It feels good to find that spark of confidence again.

The intern who guided me through the majority of the testing was very encouraging. She was very attentive to my needs and solicitous in my times of distress. She offers me water and gives me ten minutes to rest before I leave.

## *December 19*

I am trying to continue reading a self-help book. I want to take part in the exercises suggested. In doing so, I send out a message to family and friends that reads: *Hi there. Doing a self-help project. I need to ask, "What do you admire about me?" Thanks for your help with this.*

These are the replies I receive:

*I think I admire most how your own interests genuinely don't play a factor in your decisions. So selfless. I also admire how everything is in order in your world. Clean house, laundry done, on top of things…everything gets dealt with right away.* – M.S. (co-worker/ friend)

*Your energy is what I admire and your quest for always trying to learn something new. The energy you have.* – C.T. (friend)

*So it's hard to put what I love about you into words, but here goes. Your: 1) Faith/Spirituality. 2) Sincerity. 3) Kindness to all.* – T.I. (friend)

*You are one of the truest people I have ever met. Someone I have come to love and trust beyond words.* – S.W. (friend)

*How you care for everyone else. I admire that you can read when people are feeling down and do what you can to make them feel better. Personally, when I've had finals or stressful times and you plan getaways for us. Coffee dates with your friends. You have a very big and caring heart momma bear.* – J.H. (family)

*Caring. Towards family and others. Spiritual.* – P.M. (family)

*I have always admired (and mildly coveted) your amazingly diverse accomplishments. Strong academic student, excellent interpersonal skills, published author, skilled at crafts and baking, successful business owner—the list kind of goes on and on.* – A.T. (educator)

*You are a "bringer together of people."* – C.S. (friend)

These responses help me see that what people admired in me is all still there, and that I really haven't changed my values. I really needed to come to this realization. This exercise helps a great deal in improving my confidence and recognizing myself.

As I look back over this past month, I know that I'm more tolerant of being perfectly imperfect, and I like that this attitude takes some pressure off of me. I like that I have the time to be home with Blair and cherish every moment, every adventure, that we have together. I'm proud of the way I've quit comparing my life and finances to others. I like that I've been more focused on living with an attitude of gratitude. I love that cognitive limitations haven't touched my values or my beliefs— those things that are the real *me*.

## *What I have learned ...*

Are you missing reading? Audiobooks and podcasts are a wonderful way to "scratch that itch." There are lots of free apps to help you. I use the "Libby" app, which is tied to our local library. There are still so many questions I have about my brain's ability to heal. I've listened to Dr. Daniel Amen speak in a few podcasts and have found him to be both encouraging and informative. In his research, he has connected mental health issues to brain injuries. In podcasts, he discusses how researchers are finding new ways to heal the brain and resolve countless numbers of symptoms.

Be aware that you may be required to have cognitive assessments for insurance or other reasons. The testing I had to do is not a usual requirement for all claimants. However, it is important to be aware that further testing may be required to approve your claim.

Try different treatments to find what works for you. My research found the following benefits of Indian Head Massage:

- Helps prevent migraines, headaches, and back pain
- Relieves sleeplessness, restlessness, and insomnia (I can confirm that this treatment helped my sleep the afternoon, night, and for four or five days following the treatment).

- Relieves symptoms of anxiety and depression (it definitely had a calming effect on me).
- Renews energy levels
- Boosts memory capabilities (this was not noticeable for me but may help with regular treatments).

Create the highest, grandest vision possible for your life, because you become what you believe.
*Oprah Winfrey*

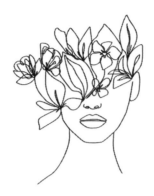

# Month 8

### (December 21, 2019–January 20, 2020)

## *December 21*

Christmas time—and I am saddened to realize that the seasonal gatherings are really challenging. Crowds and noise make me very dizzy. I am starting to let go of the negative, limiting thoughts tied to my career, my home business, time on the computer, and reading. I feel like I'm starting to realign my life to better fit my abilities and feel better about what I am able to do. Overall, I am feeling less anxious, less unbalanced, more grounded and ready to make some positive changes.

I am taking Mom around town to do a little personal and

Christmas shopping. She seems to have settled back in at the care home so nicely. I like to hear her talk about their activities and I am happy that an old friend has been picking her up for outings. I know she's making an effort to show me that I don't need to worry about her. I appreciate that. At the same time, I'm trying to show her that I'm doing better and she doesn't need to worry about me. It's that loving dance we do each time we get together.

## December 25

Christmas at Justine's. It is so good to see everyone. We enjoy a few games, and we have family pictures taken. Justine and Layne have prepared a wonderful meal for the thirteen of us. Such a fun and relaxing afternoon, and wonderful memories were made.

As seems to be the norm, I fall asleep as soon as we pull out of the driveway and I awake when we arrive home.

## December 28

Vision board day. I like the optimism of making a vision board and taking the time to dream. I have been making visions boards every December for the past five years. I post it beside my desk in my bedroom/writing area and look at it every day. I study the words I've used chosen for this upcoming year, and they include *more fun, joy, travel, enjoy more family time, continue to learn and grow, less controlling, serve others, peace and daily meditation and/or prayer.* My picture collage includes an open book with the words *write your book,* a picture of hundred-dollar bills with the words *financial abundance,* a picture of the Christmas display at the Bellagio in Las Vegas, and Jane Goodall quote I found just last week that really spoke to me: "You cannot get through a single day without having an impact on the world around you. What you do makes a difference, and you have to decide what kind of difference you want to make."

I'm happy with my completed board. I'm exhausted but feel hope for the year to come.

## *December 31*

I have decided to give up my kitchenware home business of six years. I don't feel safe enough driving to do home parties but, even more, I'm not able to be on the computer long enough to be able to do virtual parties. Trying to keep up with my little "side hustle" is just causing me too much stress and anxiety. I know I can always come back to it. It is a hard decision to make, but I have such a sense of relief now that I've made it.

For New Year's Eve, Blair and I attend a wedding dance for our friends' son. The music is loud, but I am able to find a comfortable couch in the hallway, so I sit there to visit with friends. It's important for me to set some boundaries like this so I can continue to participate in social outings. It's sometimes awkward and I feel like I am being judged by some, but it is getting easier as my friends and family have extended their understanding, and they graciously accommodate my comfort levels so I am able to be a part of these important celebrations. At the end of the night, on this New Year's Eve, I reflect on how life has changed for us, since one day back in May. It hasn't been easy, but I'm proud of how my attitude has been more positive of late. We're going to be okay.

## *January 2*

I am frustrated by trying to do mental tasks that used to be so easy! I want to just sit down to the computer and search for something without having to work hard to think of the words, or to remember what the function keys do or how to print a document! I want to read for pure enjoyment. I want to be able to go into a store without the sounds and the sights throwing me off balance. Today I've gone back a few steps in my recovery. I want to continue the momentum I've built with my positive attitude, but for today, I'm not feeling it.

## *January 3*

My father-in-law is in hospital to have a stent inserted—it was a rather sudden event. I am grateful to be able to pull out some of my medical background as we meet with doctors; I feel like I am able to talk intelligently, mostly. Even though emotional events seem to drain my energy, I am glad that in a situation that felt like an emergency, I was able to keep my energy up enough to be helpful. We are spending the night in Regina. Both Blair and I are exhausted.

## *January 4*

Driving home from the city, I am curious to know how Blair is coping with the aftermath of my stroke. I have been thinking about this for some time now, and the timing feels right to ask him my questions, here in the quiet of the car.

Me: Have I changed?
*Blair: Yes*
Me: How?
*Blair: More confused, more confrontational, anxious sometimes, some days more eager to do things — try something old, something new.*
Me: How do you feel about this new me?
*Blair: Not sure because you're not there yet.*

Me: What do you hope for me?

*Blair: Peace of mind.*

Me: Is there a part of me you'd like to not see come back?

*Blair: Don't want to see you go back to the high-stress life even though I know you liked it.*

Me: Are you still feeling like you're my caregiver?

*Blair: Sometimes. I feel like I need to remind you when you're getting overwhelmed.*

Me: What do you hope for me work-wise?

*Blair: Find something you're happy with. Be happy and not regret leaving your member relations job at the Co-op.*

Me: Are you worried about finances if I can't go back to my job?

*Blair: No, we'll be fine.*

Me: What's still on your bucket list?

*Blair: Only 50/50 on whether or not we do the Panama Canal cruise we planned before your stroke. I've done all I wanted to do.*

Me: What are some good things that have happened because of the stroke?

*Blair: You have more home time, more friend time, more hobby time.*

Me: What is the most negative aspect of the stroke?

*Blair: Answering all these questions! Not knowing what to expect one or two years down the road.*

Me: What was the scariest part of the stroke?

*Blair: Thinking that you might not come home, not be able to express yourself, end up sitting in a geriatric ward.*

Me: Do you think we're closer because of it?

*Blair: Probably. I feel like I'm more watchful of when you're getting tired.*

Me: What are you most proud of since this experience started?

*Blair: How we've come through it pretty good.*

Me: Are there old things you wish would come back?

*Blair: Not unless you want them back and they don't do damage.*

Me: Any other thoughts?

*Blair: This has been a big learning curve. Things can change in a day!*

I come away from the conversation feeling blessed to be so loved by this man. In all our years together, he has been very supportive and, most importantly, honest with me. I really respect that about him. I know and trust he always wants the best for me.

## *January 6*

My critical illness application from September 23, 2019, has been approved! I could cry. Some financial relief is on the way. *Thank you, Lord, for providing for us.*

Coincidentally, we have an appointment with a financial advisor today with the hope of bringing our investments to someone local whom we can lean on more easily when we need support or answers to questions.

Again, today mental tasks are burdensome. I want to order some pictures from Walmart. I have done it many times before my stroke, but I get in a loop of making the same mistakes on the computer and deleting my order. So frustrating! I am just going to have to walk away before this crushes me.

## January 10

My anxiety and stress levels are high again today. Am I trying to do too much? Not being able to do simple tasks is frustrating me. I want to respond differently, but this is starting to make me panic. I will book another emotional reflexology appointment—it significantly helped me before, and I am confident it will help take the edge off now.

## January 13

Some days I just want to feel fun and laughter again. Today, I am setting my intention to smile more and to look for something that feels like fun.

My intention has been fulfilled! As Blair and I are chatting over coffee, I remember a funny part of my ambulance ride on the day of my stroke. I was in the back of the ambulance, unable to speak, two IV lines in my arms, just happy to be lying down and resting, when I realized how badly I needed to pee. I was pretty sure I'd heard Blair's voice in the ambulance, so I thought maybe if I could find the word for 'pee' I could tell him. I looked up and saw the kind, familiar face of the EMT, our friends' son, but I didn't want to bother him with this need of mine to find a restroom. I started looking up to the back window of the ambulance to get a bearing of where we were on the highway. About halfway between Assiniboia and Moose Jaw is an old-style outhouse, affectionately known as "Carlson's Crapper," built and maintained by the Carlson family for anyone to use. The story has it that Dad Carlson drove his boys to hockey regularly during the winter months and there was always a need for a bathroom break before they got to their destination or back home. He built this outhouse on his land, which was central to their travels. That was a generation ago, but the place is still well maintained. The lawn around it is mowed and inside there are storage containers with magazines and toilet paper. We have stopped there only a few times, but it was a welcome place in an emergency.

There in the back of the ambulance, my thought was that we could maybe just make a quick stop. I wouldn't be long. I was sure the ambulance staff would know about Carlson's Crapper, as most locals have stopped there, or heard stories of those of us who have. I looked up again at the young man by my side. He was looking concerned. I'm sure he was wondering what I was watching for out the back of the ambulance. I worked so hard to get hold of a word to let him know my plan. I finally blurted out "Pee!" He asked if I wanted a bedpan. I realized he wasn't going to stop the ambulance nor was I going to ask this young man for a bedpan. "Sorry buddy." I remember thinking, "Love ya, but we're not going there."

Blair and I laugh almost to the point of spilling our coffee. Oh, that laugh feels good. We're going to be okay. We're going to figure this out. There are going to be lots of laughs still. I just know it.

## *January 15*

City trip today. I have an appointment with the psychologist for a review of my neuropsychological assessment. The report says I have a "mild neurocognitive disorder due to another medical condition (left hemispheric stroke), without behavioural disturbance." The psychologist tells me I have a "high cognitive reserve," meaning that all my past training isn't lost—it's still in there. That is such encouraging news for me today! I've had so many days of not being able to think through tasks that were rote before. I'm going to trust that I'll learn how to retrieve that information. There are days recently when I've had moments of clarity; for example, I explained a complex cellular structure to someone. We were both surprised to hear the number of details that I was sharing. That too was encouraging. I'm so incredibly grateful that I took the opportunity to learn when I did.

I must say, for a short time I struggle with the diagnosis, as there is still so much I'm unable to do, such as reading for any length of time, and looking at a computer screen without getting headaches, not to mention my sudden episodes of fatigue. This doesn't feel "mild"—but then again these limitations weren't part of this test.

I was happy to report to the psychologist that my insurance company accepted her report and approved my application. She was happy for me.

I slept through most of my emotional reflexology appointment. I am already feeling a decrease in anxiety. So glad I found this practitioner. She's so compassionate and so good at what she does.

## *January 16*

I hear this quote today: "A lesson learned should be a lesson shared." This really speaks to me. I'm beginning to think about the possibility, and need, to write a book that will help others navigate through the first few months after a stroke or similar brain injury. I feel these days of frustration are here to help me find resolutions and that the process will be valuable to share with others.

## *January 20*

A good day today. I feel a spark again—the start of that little flame inside of me that makes me want to try something new. I am also feeling a sense of curiosity again. The feeling is similar to reuniting with a favourite old friend. I might even feel some passion—I'm not sure what for, but it feels like things are about to change. And I am so ready for change. Ready and willing to "bend like the willow," a phrase I heard many years ago at a medical records conference. We were being prepared for a major change in the way data was going to be coded and collected. The imagery suggests that the willow tree remains strong even when it must bend to the wind. I always liked that visual reference.

## *What I have learned ...*

**What you focus on grows.** I am understanding that idea more and more. It's as easy, and as hard, as changing your attitude about how you perceive what's going on in your life. For me, I had to consciously quit thinking that we lacked finances. Instead, when those thoughts crept in, I would make a point of being grateful for our safe, comfortable home or the food in our fridge and freezer, or the warmth of our bed. The less time I spent stewing about our financial shortfalls, the more it seemed that money came our way and stayed with us longer.

I also kept hearing myself tell people what I couldn't do. I made a conscious effort to change that conversation to celebrating what I could do. I can listen to audio books and podcasts to scratch that itch I have to learn and enjoy a good story being told. I reveled in telling about the wonderful meals we'd been cooking at home. After all, with my side business, I had a wonderfully stocked kitchen of great cooking tools and really enjoyed spending time creating new dishes. I even began talking about writing a book, trusting that what I focused on would grow.

**Make positive affirmations.** They help to keep you in a clear, constructive frame of mind. We all have negative beliefs about ourselves. Making positive affirmations is a great way to change that programming in our thoughts to help us feel better about ourselves and where we are in life. Some days I need to tell myself that I'm okay and that I'm not broken. I allow myself to think, *What if I wasn't broken? What could I do? What can I do? What can I be?* I believe that all things happen for good even if that means going through a hard space to find out what that is. Some days I have to dig deep past the frustration and fear and give myself permission to be happily retired and to be grateful for the days I get to spend hanging out with Blair.

Take a moment to think about what you are currently believing about yourself. Awareness is the first step. The trick is to say these positive affirmations consistently, even if you don't believe them at first. The subconscious mind is powerful. We just need to feed it the right information—the right beliefs for our lives.

Write your affirmations in the positive, using "I am" statements. State your declaration in the present tense and include emotion words such as *enjoy, grateful for, excited about, enthusiastic about*, and *focused on*.

Here are a few of mine:

*I am strong enough.*
*I am grateful to be able to write and share my story to help others.*
*I give myself permission to be a successful, inspired writer/author/*

*speaker.* (This one is on a Post-it note on my laptop.)

*I am able to encourage, empower, and educate stroke survivors and their caregivers.*

*I am obediently following God's path and purpose for me.*

*I am compassionate.*

*I am financially abundant. Money flows to me easily, freely, and abundantly.*

*I am filled with God's love and joy to overflowing.*

*I am worthy.*

*I love and forgive myself.*

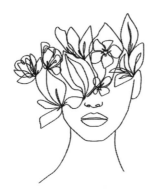

# Month 9
## (January 21–February 21, 2020)

## *January 21*

Today I speak with a prospective new employer about some part-time work. *Very* part-time. The employer is willing to wait until May in the hope that when I reach the one-year mark after my stroke, I will have regained even more cognitive function. It's such an encouraging day. Before my stroke, I entertained the thought of retiring from the Co-op to spend more time with Blair. I shared this idea with a community member who responded by asking if I would be interested in a bit of part-time work.

I liked that idea, but had assumed that this offer was off the table now because of my stroke.

My optimism about potential future employment is shadowed by doubts. I know this offer was based on knowing me as I was when I was energized and excited about working with our customers and community. Because I was so involved with the process of charitable donations, I was very much aware of projects in our surrounding areas that needed financial support and goods-in-kind. This knowledge is valuable to a new company in town that wants to quickly assimilate with the people and businesses. What better way to do that than for the company to reach out and offer to take part? Is it fair of me to let this employer assume that I still operate on that same level of energy and knowledge? I suspect that I am having more incidents of memory loss than I'm aware of, based on near-arguments with Blair. The arguments are about what I assume is his failure to share plans with me and the worsening of our communication skills, when really it may be that I just don't remember the conversations. How does that fit into a work world?

Optimism and doubt seem to walk hand in hand lately. I know I continually waver between working and not working. I'm grateful for my uplifting optimism and consciously dwell on that positive feeling while tamping down the doubt that lies just below the surface, always.

## *January 23*

This is an October 22nd kind of day. A Great Day! Life is feeling brighter than usual. Tonight is a Ladies Night Out with a few friends at the community centre across the street from our home. Supper and a movie. The perfect end to a bright day. What would I do without my friends? I treasure the constant caring and reassurance I receive from these ladies whom I can just as easily laugh with as cry with. I count myself blessed.

(This day was followed by one day of cautious optimism, one very irritable day, and two days of very low energy, when even speaking felt like too much effort.)

## *January 27*

Blair and I decide to take off on a last-minute getaway to the western town of Deadwood, South Dakota. The drive is about seven and a half hours, but great winter weather is predicted, so why not? A great hotel promotion has rooms at just forty dollars per night, so we decide to stay for three days. The town has an old gold mine we want to see if it's open during the off-season. We enjoy travelling, and this is the affordable little getaway we both need.

The drive has been so enjoyable. We are listening to a podcast on the history of Deadwood, but we lose the connection when we cross the U.S. border. We'll have to listen to the rest of it when we get back. Blair treasures historical stories. I love the way he's immersed himself in these stories of days gone by. It's fun to go to a place where you have a bit of an understanding of its past— the best way to be a tourist.

We arrive safely at this cobblestoned, friendly little town. Because it's off-season, there are very few people around, and with the mild weather, we enjoy walking to explore the community. Near our hotel, we come across an excavation site of tunnels that have been discovered under the streets. Not too much information is being shared about the site at this point, but it's exciting nonetheless.

We are relishing the guilt-free sleep ins, lazy mornings of watching TV in bed, and then explorations of the town. We take rides on the little town trolley for just a dollar. Just are cognizant of this precious time together. We need this so much. We both experience that carefree, holiday feeling we had just a year ago when we joined my cousin and her husband in Hawaii. I can feel my shoulders relax and drop. My time with Blair is quality partnership time. Neither of us is a caregiver today; we are spouses enjoying each other's company as we explore the wild west.

I'm not a real fan of ghost stories or horror movies. I just scare too easily. As we were lazily lying in bed I was sure I heard horse hooves hitting the cobblestone street just outside our window. *How fun!* I thought as I ran to the window to see them. But there were no horses. The street was empty. I asked Blair if he heard them, but he hadn't, as he was focused on a TV program. However, he did start to listen too, and we heard it again! We both ran to the window and tore back the curtains. Again, no horses. Things started to feel creepy. A car drove by and again we heard the sound. And, as we soon discovered, car tires over cobblestones sound exactly like horse hooves hitting the ground. My heart is full as we laugh together at the window.

## February 3

I am still trying to test how much time I can tolerate on the laptop, to try to avoid getting the inevitable headache. Today, over a four-hour stretch, I probably looked at the screen intermittently for about two hours. So far, this four-hour test seems like it went well.

## February 4

Extreme headache today. By noon, I had to take Tylenol and go back to bed. Maybe too much time in front of the screen yesterday. But I won't give up. I will monitor my screen time more carefully. Maybe one hour at a stretch is enough for now. I've tried repeatedly to find out why the onset of my headaches is so delayed. It would be much easier to test my limits if the headache started while I'm on the computer, so I would know when it is time to quit.

## *February 5*

Back when I had my follow-up visit with the surgeon, he mentioned that people are more prone to experience sleep apnea after a stroke, and he recommended that I take part in a sleep study. Sleep apnea is a condition in which a person stops breathing repeatedly during sleep; the breathing stops because the airway collapses and prevents air from getting into the lungs. Sleep patterns are disrupted, resulting in excessive sleepiness or fatigue during the day. Tonight and tomorrow night I will do a home sleep study and will expect results in two to three weeks.

The process was pretty easy, and the instructions were very easy. The equipment monitored my breathing patterns, oxygen levels, and heart rate. A microphone monitored snoring, a nasal cannula measured airflow, and an effort belt around my chest measured chest expansion and contraction with each breath. As well, a finger probe measured the percentage of oxygen in my blood and recorded my heart rate. This sounds a bit complicated and unwieldy, but it wasn't. I used the equipment for two nights and then took it all back to have the data interpreted.

## *February 14*

Not only is this Valentine's Day, it's also Justine's 29th birthday, so we have supper out to celebrate with her. I always enjoy time with our families. Conversations continue to create brain fatigue, but for the short time we're together I try to just enjoy the togetherness. I have to admit that my filters still seem unstable and I'm saying things that I would have held back in the past. I think this is changing my relationship with some family members. It's not a good or bad thing, just a thing.

## *February 20*

Blair's father is in hospital to have a pacemaker inserted. The procedure seems to have gone well. We leave the hospital when other family members come to visit. Before we get home, we receive a call that a Code Blue was called, so we race back to Regina.

He was successfully resuscitated and barely remembers the incident other than he had an incredible need to yawn, and that was the last thing he remembered.

I am so grateful that he was in good hands and in the hospital when it happened. Consistent with any of my emotional episodes, I have significant fatigue and I need to sleep on the way home.

## *February 21*

We are relieved to find out that Blair's dad rested comfortably for the rest of the evening. It was determined that the episode had been caused by a faulty pacemaker setting, and it had been corrected. He is able to return home today. Coincidentally, I receive good health news too. I do not have sleep apnea!

## *What I have learned ...*

**Learn about the role of diet in your brain health.**
There is so much we can do to help our brain just by
paying attention to the food we eat. The brain uses about
20 to 30 percent of our energy intake. Eating a diet that
contains brain-healthy nutrients is essential for good
brain health.

The following are some brain-healthy foods you can add
to your diet. Or take a moment now and celebrate the
good you're already doing!

- Fatty fish (tuna, herring, sardines) are a high
  source of omega-3 fatty acids, a building block
  for the brain. Omega-3 helps sharpen memory
  and improve mood. It may also protect your brain
  against cognitive decline.
- Blueberries are rich in antioxidants and also have
  an anti-inflammatory property. They may delay
  brain aging and improve memory.
- Turmeric has curcumin as its active ingredient.
  Curcumin has been shown to cross the blood-brain
  barrier to benefit the brain cells with improved
  memory, ease of depression and new brain cell
  growth. You can buy curcumin as a supplement,
  as the percentage available in turmeric is quite low.
- Broccoli also has antioxidants which may help

protect the brain against damage. Broccoli is also very high in Vitamin K. Some studies link Vitamin K to better memory and cognitive status.

- Dark chocolate is packed with brain-boosting compounds such as flavonoids (antioxidant, anti-inflammatory, and immune-boosting), caffeine, and antioxidants (Halleluia!). According to research, chocolate is also a mood booster.
- Some studies show that sage enhances memory.

**Listen to your thoughts about other people.** If they are negative thoughts, stop them and replace them with thoughts of what you appreciate about that person. I find this particularly helpful as our family relationships are changing. If my filters are less effective at keeping my thoughts to myself, I want to be sharing positive thoughts. This all takes practice, but is worth the effort.

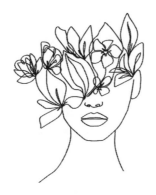

# Month 10
### (February 22–March 20, 2020)

## *February 22*

I'm still experiencing reduced filters (speaking my mind more than I used to). I'm working on this change in my personality—or, maybe, am I using this change as an opportunity to speak out more freely? I am certainly not always getting positive reactions to this change in me. Part of me feels bad, but part of me feels stronger. Did holding things in contribute to stress? Maybe even to stroke?

## *February 25*

A friend recently reached out and shared with me the benefits of 'grounding.' She described to me the health benefits of exposing yourself to the ions that are most beneficial to your body's health. This is recommended for healing parts of the body and has also shown to have benefit for some cancer patients.

We all know how much better we feel when we are vacationing on a beach. Is it the slower pace that makes us feel better? Or is it that we are taking in the health benefits of sunshine (Vitamin D)? Or is it the fact that our feet are out of shoes, and instead of walking on cement, we are walking on the grass and in the sand? It's proven that standing with your bare feet on the ground changes the ionization of your body. Similarly, a grounding sheet—which has a ground wire that you can feed out your window and stick in the ground or you can plug it into the ground hole of your electrical socket (that little third hole that is above or below the two holes for your two-prong plug)—has the same effect of changing the ionization of the body.

I'm always curious and am open to trying therapies that don't have any indication of being harmful. So today is the first day with the grounding sheet that I ordered online. This black sheet, with small holes through it, lies on top of a fitted sheet, and you sleep directly on it. You can order it to fit your mattress size. The material of the grounding sheet takes a little getting used to, as it has a vinyl-like feel. The wire to the ground hole of the socket is at the head of the bed, so I'm feeling overly cautious about inadvertently pulling the wire out if my arms or pillows touch it during the night. (That never did happen, though.)

I have a watch that monitors my sleep patterns, and for all my first week of sleeping on the sheet, the watch shows that I have had a dramatic increase in REM sleep each night. I am feeling more rested and I have more clarity in my thoughts. I am still experiencing "brain crashes" when I try to read too much, or have too much screen time, too much conversation, or am in a very emotional state.

## February 27

I sincerely believe I have been grieving—experiencing real grief—from the loss of the ability to read for long periods. I cannot read long enough to reach that point where I've stepped into the world the author has created or where I can feel the depth of everything that the characters are experiencing. I can no longer read an educational piece and feel the satisfaction of the "aha moment"—that moment when what you're reading makes such clear sense and you know you can apply the information in your life or bring clarity and understanding to something you've been curious about. My comprehension and reading ability last only about twenty minutes. I am so frustrated and bereft by this. But, today I celebrate finally finishing a novel that I started before my stroke! A novel that formerly would have been a weekend read has taken me nine months to complete. Reading is now a very different experience, much less enjoyable, but I'm stubborn and I wanted to enjoy the intrigue of the twisted plot and turn that last page. Mission accomplished! Turning another "I can't" to an "I can!"

## *March 13*

To avoid letting my world shrink to daily inventories of what I can and can't do, I know that it's important to keep my heart open to helping others. Today I have the opportunity to volunteer for a shift on the phones for a local fundraiser. All I need to do is take down names, phone numbers, and credit card info from people wanting to buy tickets. It feels quite enjoyable. I feel good to be giving back to a community that has always been supportive of Blair and I. Later I experience a significant headache and fatigue. I awaken at 2 a.m. with a severe headache.

Today we experience the stunning news release stating

that all Assiniboia recreation facilities are being closed today due to Covid-19. As we understand it, it's a virus that began in Wuhan City, China, and is spreading quickly, worldwide. Those most at risk, we are told, are the elderly and the very young. I realize that I have to share this with Mom and will need to make sure she is staying safe and maybe even staying put in her care home until we know more.

## *March 14*

Saskatchewan has its first confirmed Covid-19 case. This is concerning—a virus that originated in China is now here, in North America. In our province! We are hearing lots of speculation about whether it was an intentional form of germ warfare or simply a new strain of an old virus that is now more virulent. Countless questions, countless opinions. We are desperate for facts.

## *March 15*

Because Covid-19 is appearing in greater numbers in Saskatchewan, we are following the direction of health care experts and self-quarantining. Blair's cancer and my stroke put us at higher risk. Already our local grocery stores are encouraging people to stay home and to email in their grocery orders instead, with free delivery.

I know this sounds terribly selfish, but I actually appreciate not having to go into stores, with all their visual and audio stimulation that affects me so negatively. Being in any store environment still makes me physically uncomfortable, so having a reason to spend more time at home is actually fine with me. Also, I find that I'm okay with not being out and having conversations that can have a noticeable effect on my brain. I am experiencing such conflicting feelings—I know that so many people are going to struggle with isolation and quarantine, and everything is so uncertain. I also recognize the huge importance of staying quarantined and doing what we can to remain safe from this potentially deadly strain. Blair has survived his battle with cancer; I do not want to lose him to a virus!

## *March 16*

Prairie Villa, Mom's care home, is locked down to keep their residents safe. I have to say this makes me feel a little panicked; it hits hard when I truly recognize that this virus is *real*. I wonder, with Mom's advancing dementia, if she's able to understand what is going on. We are told that we can visit with the residents through their bedroom window, which offers some comfort. Thankfully we can continue to chat via phone. I know these safety measures are there to protect this vulnerable group in our community.

## *March 17*

Once again, I appreciate the value of being members of a small community. Things have been shut down only a few days and already friends are offering to bring groceries or run errands for us so we can "stay home, stay safe."

The pandemic is foremost on everyone's mind. Some huge life changes are happening, and people are experiencing panic and fear. I feel that I've already been living in panic and fear for ten months and I'm just starting to figure my way through it. Having done the work already for this long has actually, surprisingly, made the announcement of Covid-19 just another blip on my personal radar because I had coping skills already in place. My prayer is that those who have never experienced a major, traumatic life event can find coping skills quickly that will help them manage their fear and feelings of uncertainty.

## *What I have learned ...*

**Try this exercise to decrease anxiety.** Whether it's a pandemic or any other life event that is causing anxiety, here is an exercise that will keep everything in perspective. When anxious thoughts are running through your mind, write them down. It might look like this:

- "I'm going to die. My kids are going to die!"
- "I can't work. I have no income! I'm going to be bankrupt!"
- "I'm so scared. Is this literally going to be the end of the world?"

Now, are these thoughts/statements *true*? Do a little research; it'll make you feel better.

- Why are you worrying about death right now? What are some statistics about death? Is the death rate low in your area? Check the rates for the age groups that apply to you or your family.
- Are there other work options that will make you feel safer? Working from home? Different job? When you feel that you're in a financial crisis, it's a good time to look at your spending habits. Living through a pandemic makes you realize that you *can* live without movies, pub nights with friends, vacations to faraway destinations. If you

can cut back enough to reduce your stress, even for a short time or even a year or two, you will find your financial footing again. Don't hesitate to reach out for help from financial advisors. They are wonderful at helping you see the truth of your situation rather than live in fear.

- No matter the gravity of the situation, like the pandemic, really think about it. Is it the end of the world? Who knows? If it were, is there anything you can do to change it? Instead of spending your days in fear, open your heart and eyes to the blessings in your life. You have so much to be grateful for. This is a great time to hold firm to your faith, your higher power, your love for one another.

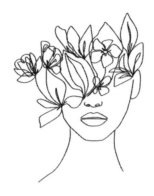

# Month 11
## (March 21-April 20, 2020)

### *March 27*

Following my endarterectomy surgery on May 27, 2019 (about a week after my stroke), I was left with significant numbness in my left lower gum as well as my left jaw all the way down to my collarbone and as far forward as my chin. For years, I've had a space between two teeth on the back left side of my mouth that always seems to get food caught in it. The sensation of fullness around those back teeth was a convenient reminder to floss regularly. It's very odd to not have that sensation anymore and for flossing to become a more conscious routine. However, today, while flossing my teeth, I noticed that feeling is returning to my left lower jaw and gum while the area under my chin is still numb. I almost want to celebrate that sensation of food in my teeth again. I might even go grab a stick of celery to chew on just to feel that annoying fullness and the need to go and floss because I have to, and not just because I know I should.

It's been ten months since my stroke, and I'm still experiencing subtle changes and improvements like this. I'm also living with headaches, fatigue, and occasional brain fog—these seem to be the constants that remind me that I've still got healing to do.

Several of the medical professionals tell me that any cognitive impairments I still have at the one-year mark will be what I'm left with. Other professionals tell me the benchmark is two years. My hope is that healing will continue, and I'll arrive at the day I can say, "Remember when … I struggled with headaches, with the inability to read and comprehend, with unpredictable fatigue, with the rollercoaster of emotions, with having to limit my time in front of a computer screen?"

I've learned so many ways to cope, and when I'm in a good space, they work so well to keep me happy and content. But when I don't make walking a priority, or if I get lax in taking supplements that keep my brain functioning optimally, or when I fall off the low-carb wagon, I experience a wave of frustration and despair. I don't like that I take out my frustrations on friends and family, especially Blair. I don't like me when that happens.

When I'm in the depths of these lows, I don't even see that I'm there until something happens that makes me embarrassed to see how poorly I'm coping. At that point, I mentally take time to reset and get back on track.

Those waves aren't as deep or as often now as they were. I'm grateful for that. I'm grateful that I continue to find ways to make life better for myself. I'm grateful that friends and family are respectful of the boundaries I need to set with regard to length of time engaging in group conversations, with planning a quiet space to retreat to if the environment I'm in gets too overwhelming, and with my even having to say "no" to attending an event at all.

## *April 4*

I am still enjoying little projects that keep my mind busy and fill my days. I thrive on the feeling of completion and the satisfaction of seeing a finished project. I'm able to stitch for an hour or so at a sitting and enjoy doing puzzles, but for shorter periods of time before the visual disturbance makes it impossible to continue. Doing both activities in the same day fatigues my brain, but today I push that envelope. I am taking frequent naps of twenty minutes to an hour this afternoon, as my brain requires—no, demands—that I rest.

Covid-19 stats to date: 14,000 cases in Canada; 300,000 cases in the U.S. These numbers are quickly climbing all around the globe. Crafting and puzzling distract me from dwelling on the panic and fear created by this virus that has become a pandemic.

As always, I am grateful that Mom is in a safe place. I wonder, if this virus hits our community, if Jared and Justine will be exposed to something that will affect their bodies, in this child-bearing stage of life they are in. Will my dad, and Blair's mom and dad, understand the seriousness of what's happening and stay safe? They aren't on social media to see these daily numbers increasing so quickly, but it is being covered more and more on TV now. *Lord, please wrap us in Your loving arms and protect us from the virus. Please replace our worry and fear with peace. Please help us to trust that You are in control. In Jesus' name I pray. Amen*

## *April 8*

Covid-19 stats on cases to date: World—1.5 million; U.S.—430,000; and Canada—19,000. Due to the virus, some churches are closing down and are live-streaming their services instead. I see that my favourite pastor, Pastor

Mark, is leading a church in Ontario and he has already moved his services to live-streaming. I started attending an online Bible Study with Pastor Mark today. So good to see this familiar face and to learn with him again. He has such a fun, easy way of sharing The Message.

It's been years since I've been part of a Bible study and I miss it. I know how good it is for my soul and I love looking deeper into the meaning of the scriptures.

A local church has been broadcasting their service for quite some time and I enjoy tuning into that. Sadly, our attendance at an in-person service has been sporadic since Blair's cancer diagnosis. The church we had been attending is about a fifty-kilometre drive away. When Blair was going through surgery and treatments, we just didn't have the energy nor were we awake early enough to make the drive, so I occasionally attended a few different church services here in town. I am aware that our church family and other groups of believers I'm involved with lift us up and keep us in their prayers.

I'm so grateful to have this connection with Pastor Mark again. Today, I'm reminded that even though there are things that I've lost due to the stroke, my faith isn't one of them.

## *April 9*

Mom's left arm has been swelling over the past few days. She has an appointment in Moose Jaw for a Doppler ultrasound to check blood flow. I drive, with just Mom in the car. I haven't driven this far in almost a year. I sleep while Mom has her ultrasound, as I am very brain-tired. We are told that Mom has small clots on her pacemaker leads, and she is given a new prescription to address the problem. Due to Covid, Mom will have to stay isolated in her room at her residence for fourteen days and then see a doctor after fourteen days for follow-up, followed by another fourteen days of isolation. (Near the end of Mom's isolation period, she confided in me that she felt bad that everyone in her residence had to be locked down because of her trip to the doctor. I hadn't realized that she didn't understand that Covid-19 was the culprit to the rules and I felt so sorry that she was blaming herself. It took a fair amount of explaining and repeating that Covid really was the reason and not her. By the time I left, she seemed to be reassured that she really wasn't to blame. It was good to see her relax, knowing she wasn't the cause of this new protocol.)

## *April 11*

I don't wake up until 11 a.m. I am still brain-tired since driving to Moose Jaw two days ago. I start a puzzle to try to distract myself from this brain-fog feeling.

Covid case stats: World–1.8 million; U.S.–535,000; Canada–almost 24,000 cases.

The catch phrase these days is "Stay home, stay safe." Blair and I rarely watch the news, but have tuned in a little more to see the daily Covid stats. We are thankful to be in a position such that choosing to stay home doesn't really change our lifestyle much. In fact, we just commented how grateful we are for a full freezer and for the creativeness with food that our moms taught us so we can plan meals that are fun and interesting with the food we already have on hand.

I've been trying to make myself go out and be more social because I fear losing those skills. I have some "coffee-time friends" who listen to my worries and struggles, celebrate my successes, and confide in me about what is going on in their lives. I love that these relationships have stayed solid. I love that even though we are cautioned to keep a distance from one another and limit exposure to crowds, this core group of friends are still there, constant and caring. What would I do without them in my world? I can live without crowds, and shopping, and even trips to the city for services or medical appointments, but it would be a sad space to be in without my friends' camaraderie.

Our in-person medical appointments are starting to switch to phone appointments, which I'm really appreciating. No more travel to the cities, with the related expenses, and no more daylong outings for a twenty-minute appointment. More time for puzzling, for crafting, for cooking.

My only wish is that our kids were in occupations that would allow them to "stay home, stay safe." In his town maintenance job, Jared works mostly outside, and other than attending council meetings, he isn't required to work with groups of people. Justine, on the other hand, spends her days helping customers with their medication reviews and questions. Businesses are starting to implement safety measures such as putting lines on the floor to keep people conscious of safe distancing, and putting up plexiglass barriers between workers and customers. Some businesses are even closing their doors to public traffic and instead are encouraging curbside pick-up. It sounds like Justine's workplace will be implementing this. I am glad for her. This feels safer.

I often think of how much extra work this would have created had I still been at work. So many safety issues for the staff, so many events to be cancelled, so many new protocols for our retail stores. I keep them in my prayers as all the retail locations I worked with are now classified as essential services and will remain open.

I'm excited that the activity worker in Dad's long-term care facility has arranged for video chats on Mondays. This is wonderful for us, and so good for his mental health—heck, for the mental health of *all* of us. In Ontario, where he resides, a designated family member is allowed to go into the facility to help with care. I have to say, this makes me anxious because I think the residents may have increased exposure. At this time, in Ontario, shopping is less restricted, and people aren't wearing masks in public like we are. But on the other hand, it's so nice for Dad to have my sister there to visit with.

I think, for the elderly, comprehending the impact of the pandemic is overwhelming and frightening. I wish I could go in and be with Mom and assure her she is safe. She and I have phone chats, and when it's not too cold out, I will stand outside her window while we talk on the phone. The activity worker in Mom's facility has amped up their scheduled activities to keep them entertained.

We are quite content to be at home, but there are days I miss friends from afar. Once I was able to figure out video chatting, I probably have connected more with them than I have in years.

We've created a safe cocoon here. Because Jared and Justine are exposed to the public, we all agree that visiting in person right now is probably not a good idea. We trust that this will be short-lived and we'll get back to seeing them face to face and exchanging hugs again soon.

We learned to pivot when Blair was diagnosed with cancer and when I had my stroke. It's almost as though these life experiences have better equipped us to pivot again. My heart goes out to the younger generation who haven't yet experienced a major life event. They haven't yet had the opportunity to live through something challenging and know that it will end. For those with young children, the pivot is huge. Already businesses are talking about staff working from home and in some provinces even talking about closing schools.

This pandemic is a life-changing event that will teach us how to pivot; how to build on skills we may not have had to use such as: cooking, becoming more tech savvy, working from home, home schooling, coping with fear and anxiety, appreciating relationships and personal contact, valuing feeling safe, and being grateful for all those people whom we now have given the title of "Essential Workers"—those who continue to work at the risk of their own personal safety. *Lord, please bless us with peace right now. There is so much fear. Please give us wisdom to do what we need to do to stop the spread of this virus. Please watch over every essential worker and keep them out of harm's way. Please be with the people who have contracted the virus and heal their bodies. Please be with the families of those who have succumbed to*

*Covid 19 and comfort them. Lord, so much to ask for. I know You are big enough and that You hear my prayers. In Jesus' name I pray. Amen*

## April 17

I know I have wavered about this, but I have resigned myself to the fact that I won't be returning to my job at the Co-op. I'm not even sure I can put together a few "good days" in a row on a regular basis to feel confident about applying for a position elsewhere. At this point, I'm not even sure I could do the other part-time job that was offered to me. I want to be able to celebrate being able to say I've retired but honestly, I've never been without a job and it's a little terrifying.

Today I submitted my application for Canada Pension Plan (CPP) Disability. I understand it will take four to six months to process. I called my group insurance provider to advise them that I've taken this first step as recommended in the CPP Disability application. I was surprised to find out that normally the Group Insurance Company would initiate the application. I apologized for jumping the gun but know that with a four-to-six-month wait on this application that I will be left with no income for three to five months. I already wish I would have applied earlier, but paperwork is so hard to work through and I've been dreading the task. Would my group insurance company have started the process earlier had Covid not happened? I'm not sure. I'm just hopeful that we can stretch our finances. Anticipating the further reduction of income until we have heard a decision, we have prepaid some bills as we were able to. Our plan, if the CPP Disability is denied, is for me to start withdrawing my regular CPP benefits early—I'm now 61. Had I already started receiving my CPP benefits, I wouldn't be eligible for CPP Disability. I feel like we're playing a financial game and it hurts my head just to figure out what to do and when.

*Lord, I pray that you'll put this application in the hands of the people who will guide us through this process more easily. Please help us be good stewards of the money you've blessed us with. Please keep our hearts grateful and Lord, please help me to see that abundance isn't about money. We have so much to be thankful for.*

## *What I have learned ...*

**Learn about CPP Disability Benefits.** It's hard to know when to apply for CPP Disability. You want to believe that tasks will get easier, that you won't always feels so limited, that you'll get back to the old you and the old job, but, in reality, you need to consider your financial future.

Prepare to give the process lots of time. In the end, my application took seven months to approve. This could be because Covid affected so many jobs, including people transitioning to working from home, or delays in mail delivery and processing paperwork.

I found that once my application was approved, I was encouraged to take training if I felt I could work in another career. There is a set gross income you are allowed to earn without affecting your benefits. For the year I was first approved, it was $5,900 per year. I was encouraged by this. I feel that, after Covid, I might want to find some part-time work or maybe even try to work my home business again. Unlike the insurance coverage on our line of credit, which threatens to terminate coverage if I have any income at all, CPP encourages some back-to-work efforts.

One CPP rep told me that if I want to try to go back to work, but then find that I'm unable to do so, that my coverage will be reinstated without the long application process that I started with.

If you have access to a financial advisor, this would be a great time to have a discussion and receive some guidance.

**Find coping strategies for anxiety.** My anxiety was worse after my stroke. Add a pandemic to the normal stressors of life and we can all use some coping strategies for our anxiety. Here are a few I found helpful:

- Watch a funny video—laughter really is the best medicine.
- Eat well-balanced meals and avoid sugar.
- Limit alcohol and caffeine, which can aggravate anxiety and trigger panic attacks.
- Get enough sleep (see tips on how to get a good night's sleep in Chapter 5).
- Exercise daily to help you feel good and maintain your health—remember that any activity that increases your heart rate and requires you to breathe more often will bring extra oxygen to your brain, and that's a good thing!
- Take deep breaths—inhale slowly and deeply through your nose. Keep your shoulders relaxed. Exhale slowly through your mouth with lips pursed and jaw relaxed. Repeat until you feel more relaxed. Deep breathing counteracts the fight or

flight stress reaction.

- Count to 10 slowly. Mostly, this will help bring your attention to the present moment.
- Practice the 5-4-3-2-1 Grounding Technique— This will help manage your anxiety by anchoring yourself in the present. Start by looking for 5 things you can see; become aware of 4 things you can touch; acknowledge 3 things you can hear; notice 2 things you can smell; then, become aware of 1 thing you can taste.
- Use meditation, especially sleep meditation. Not only does it improve sleep, you may experience the following outcomes: waking rested and calm, fewer headaches, lower blood pressure, reduced memory loss, and relief from depression and anxiety.
- Turn to prayer. Remember where your strength lies.

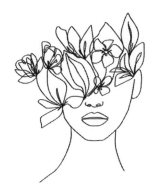

# Month 12
## (April 21-May 20, 2020)

## *April 22*

It's now been eleven months since my stroke. Blair and I have been self-isolating due to Covid-19 for six weeks. The first couple weeks were challenging, and our condo space seemed small. When the weather permitted, we opened windows—just hearing the daily noises of life outside our four walls helped us to feel better. We have a nice routine for grocery and drinking water deliveries. Going into stores is still an uncomfortable experience for my head since the stroke – too many colours, too much noise, too much conversation when I run into people I know. With all this stimulation, I start to lose my words before long, I begin to feel off balance and then either visual disturbances (like looking through a kaleidoscope) or headaches set in. I'm so happy to have the excuse to have groceries delivered.

It's Wednesday today—a great day for us, as it's the one day of the week when we have activities planned, and we so look forward to it. Daily, we keep ourselves occupied with puzzles, or stitching, or watching TV, but on Wednesdays we interact with the outside world. Our normal schedule for the day is: 2:15–video conference with Dad, organized by his nursing home activity worker; 4:30–online Bible study; 6:00–*Survivor* on TV; 7:00–online bingo put on by our town recreation manager; 8:30–online trivia game.

Today, we add to our schedule a stop at Mom's care home to drop off twenty-four mask extenders I've made for the nurses (I used plastic canvas and decorated them with colourful yarn), and a quick trip to my in-laws' home to deliver some meat they had ordered, and then a trip to try out our metal detecting skills. Such a beautiful day for a drive.

Our activities start around 1:20 p.m. with a call that our bulk order of bacon and eggs, along with the in-laws' meat order, is ready for pick-up. We quickly gather up the metal detector and the mask extenders, and we put the cooler in the vehicle. We are just driving away when Blair remembers he's forgotten to put in his dental plate with his artificial tooth, so he heads back inside and I carry on to pick up the food. I drop off our food back at the house and Blair takes it in to put in the fridge/freezer while I run up to Mom's for a quick "Hello" through the window and show her the mask extenders I've made for the staff. Our visit is short because I feel like Blair and I have so much yet to do. It's good to see her—she is such a loving woman, and she has so much caring and worry in her heart for my recovery since the stroke. I go around to the front door and buzz for a staff member to take my drop-off of mask extenders.

Blair is waiting for me when I return home. He jumps in, we drive to pick up the mail and then he takes over the wheel. The mail consists of just another insurance form for him to complete for his disability insurance. We are heading out of town and enjoying the freedom of being outside and on the road. The sun is shining, and it's good to see the wildlife. Even though it's now April, a few combines are finishing last year's harvest. Tufts of green are beginning to show on the edges of the road.

It's now 2:15 and my phone rings with the invitation to join Dad's video chat. My sister and niece are also on the chat and for a short time our daughter is able to join in. I am happy to catch up with everyone. Dad struggles to understand what is going on in the world as we compare local stories but seems to enjoy being part of the conversation. His activity worker very kindly explains things to him, and she shows us projects that she and Dad have been working on.

We've arrived at the in-laws' so it's time for me to say goodbye on the video call. I am already looking forward to seeing everyone again next week.

We pull into the parking lot of the seniors' housing complex and see four chairs strategically placed on the gravel for our visit. Blair parks the vehicle in a way that will block us from the wind. My mother-in-law brings out coffee and Blair's favourite baked treat—matrimonial cake. (Outside of Saskatchewan, this dessert is known as date squares.) We do our best to keep our distance and enjoy the visit. It's good to see them and know that they are doing well.

The plan was to next head to the farm we once owned, but we realize when we check the time that our son is already off work and we haven't yet seen the new little puppies at his house, born just this past week. Again, we keep our distance as best we can (sadly, no hugs) as Jared directs us to the room the puppies are in. Five adorable little black and white pups are soundly asleep. We wait patiently for one to stir so we can pick it up. I'm not much of a pet person, but this little creature has cuddled right into my arms and has fallen back to sleep. His face is on my chest and he stirs, licks my skin, and falls back to sleep. Another puppy makes a few tiny sounds and signals the need to be cuddled. Blair obliges. Our son shares with pride that the momma dog, Bella, has done very well in caring for her new brood. Time to put the puppies back down and say our hug-less goodbyes. My heart aches a bit each time we see the kids but can't hold them, even for a short time.

Off to our next adventure—we found the metal detector on a local buy-and-sell site this winter and with the permission of the current owner of our old farm, we are excited to see what we can find. We had sold the home quarter in 2009 when we struggled to financially recover from BSE (Mad Cow Disease) which caused not only the cattle prices to drop dramatically but also to reduce our ability to sell our cattle. Even though Blair and I were both working full-time off the farm, we couldn't gain any ground. Our kids had indicated they were not interested in farming, so we made the incredibly tough decision to sell. The previous generations recovered from their hard times, kept the homestead going—and yet we were the generation that failed to make it through.

Pulling into the yard evokes a flood of mixed emotions. It's home but it's not. The grass is overgrown except for in the yard in front of the house. I think this must be hard on Blair's heart to be back and see the changes. This is the farm that had been in his family for generations.

I know how bad the ticks get in the spring, so I have come armed with a repellent spray. I spray Blair down, trying to get the spray on his clothing rather than his skin. He returns the favour and sprays down my clothes. I ask him to spray an arc over my head but instead he sprays it directly onto my hair. I don't know why, but this triggers anxiety, and I feel it welling up inside of me. It is that too-familiar feeling of quivering, starting at my very core. I feel like if I were a runner, I'd start running to get rid of this extra internal energy. Instead, we head over to the clothesline where our son told us he buried a jar of coins as a child, hoping it would grow into a money tree. Our hope is that the metal detector will pick up the metal lid on the jar.

I had watched some YouTube videos on the use of this detecting tool—like how to angle the head of the detector, what the buttons on the readout mean, and so on. My intention was to share some of the information with Blair, but it's coming out in an angry and demeaning way. The dialogue in my head is, "He's walking too fast, he's breathing too loud." I hate this!! It's been such a good day, and now this is happening. With the detector, we first find a piece of heavy wire and then an old pair of fencing pliers. These were pretty exciting finds. Although my patience is almost non-existent, I hang in there, and we find an old shovel head welded to an iron pipe that Blair remembered making as a young adult. It wasn't even in the dirt—just buried in the overgrown grass. After that we find that our "hits" are in areas where the ground is just too frozen to dig. The smell of the repellent on my head is becoming overwhelming and nauseating. I just want to go home so I can wash it off. We agree that we'll come back when the ground has thawed. My words are louder and angrier than I want them to be but I can't seem to calm down. Best that I just stay quiet. I keep the window partly opened on the drive home. The smell is too much. I think to myself that Blair has survived seven years of cancer, but can his soul survive my words? The trip home is long, although I try to think of things to be grateful for that will override the quiver still inside of me. I'm grateful for the sunshine, for the time outside of the house, for our visit with Dad and my in-laws, for our kids and their good health. *Lord, that You will never forsake us or leave us.*

As we pull into our parking spot at home, I can't even wait for the car to get aligned before I ask Blair if he can let me out. I head up the stairs and directly into the tub. While there is only an inch or two of water in the bottom I get in and lie back to wash my hair. I try to discern whether the nausea is from the spray or from my nervous state. It doesn't matter. I know I'm okay. I just need to breathe. Although I'm still not able to read like I used to, I do find that even reading a few pages at a time helps to calm me, distract me, while I try to self-soothe. I always have a book by the tub and read what I can. After an hour of soaking, I feel calmer—regretful that I've put Blair through this again—but calmer.

*Survivor* is about to begin so I grab a glass of water and settle onto the couch. Blair says he's tired and is going to lie down. This isn't unusual after an outing, but today I don't know if he's actually tired or just feels safer retiring to the bedroom. He isn't gone very long and then remembers that we wanted to separate out the bulk box of bacon into smaller packages. He asks how many pieces he should put in each pack. I suggest that twelve would be good. He shows me what twelve in a bag looks like to see if that's enough. I see that the bacon isn't lying flat in the bag and the quiver begins again. I ask him to leave it for me to do because I'm afraid of my own words. I don't want the "bully" in me to come out. I don't like or appreciate this new, residual manifestation from the stroke.

Blair must feel safe enough to stay in my presence because he settles into his chair as I play online bingo on the couch. He joins me for the online trivia game, and that goes well. We both have some good guesses and even a few chuckles.

I'm tired. Although it's been a day of fun activities, there have been too many anxious episodes, and I'm ready for bed. As I get up, I see the box of bacon on the counter and I'm in a bad mood again. This post-stroke lack of tolerance and mean personality are occurring far too often for my liking, and I hate what this must be doing to Blair's self-esteem. I pray that he's able to know that I'm not angry at him and that he's done nothing wrong. Blair comes to help open the bags and we get it packaged up as quickly as possible. We are both beat!

But sleep just isn't happening. I can't stop my brain, my thoughts of regret, flickers of anger, and the replaying of my hurtful words and attitude today. By 2 a.m. I have a headache worthy of Tylenol and by 3 a.m., I'm finally able to sleep.

## April 23

A day like yesterday isn't new to us since the stroke. With the busyness, even though they are all enjoyable events, comes the roller coaster of emotions and attitudes that range from loving to mean and bitter.

We take each day as a new one and spend the morning enjoying coffee and a game of crib. The sun is warm today so we sit on the balcony and enjoy the fresh air. I apologize for yesterday. I love him so much and don't want to hurt his soul like I'm sure I have. He shrugs it off and we carry on. Today is a "good" day.

I sleep a lot throughout the day and conclude that, as fun as our Wednesdays are, I need to cut some activities out. The Bible study is recorded so I will watch it on another day. Even though the Wednesday events are fun things to do, they are just too much.

## April 28

I have lunch with the Co-op's Human Resources Manager today. We know that my disability benefits will come to an end next month. I ask if there is a possibility of taking a leave in the hope that my cognitive abilities will improve. Unfortunately, that's not an option. However, she says she will check to see if I could have my pension plan waiting period waived if I came back in a different capacity. After much discussion, by the end of our conversation I decide to not return to work. I am aware that I've made this decision repeatedly but then convince myself that maybe

I could manage to return in some capacity. I know I can no longer do my job and now feel a sense of acceptance.

## *May 1*

Yesterday I received my Life Insurance Policy Statement. I'd paid my annual premium last month but noticed on the statement that I have Premium Waiver. I called our insurance agent and his office sent me the forms to complete to apply for the waiver. It was several pages long and daunting, so I knew to leave it until this morning when my mind is fresh.

I sit down early to begin filling out the forms. I am very pleased with how clear my thoughts are, but by the end of page six the mental processing is much harder. I push on and fill out the consent pages and call the doctor's office to request completion of the Physician's Report. My next call is to my workplace to request the Human Resources Manager fill out the Employer Certificate. I struggle to find words. She is very understanding, and we agree that I will forward the email from the insurer with all the forms, and she will select the ones she needs and fill them out. Thankfully, I have completed all that I need to for the day. It took me about an hour and a half. I struggle with mental fatigue for the rest of the day, but feel proud of getting this task done.

## *May 2*

I had registered for an online women's conference. Several speakers in the line-up were appealing to me and the cost was only forty dollars. It ran a full day and I knew that would be far too long to watch on the computer so I set myself up with a headset so I could listen and stitch mask extenders.

The speakers were wonderful! The intention was to motivate women to have courage during this time of pandemic. The exercises helped us to identify fears and coping strategies around life at home during the Covid lockdown. We began by checking in on our current mindset. Was it fixed or was it in a growth state? How could we change our current mindset to get to where we want to be? We identified fears and made our own plan of how to overcome them.

My focus was on fears that weren't related to Covid; they were around not returning to work. We heard about focusing not on what we can't do but rather on what we *can* do.

As I listened while stitching intently, I stopped to make notes on comments that caught my attention such as: *Help someone else—you were born to do something special in your life* and *Uncover your gifts and use them to serve others.* And finally, *Of the things you want to do, do just one.* For me, I have discovered over time, that 'one thing' was to write a book. Just a few pages at a time if necessary. It *will* get done.

Another speaker offered the thought that your life will become a direct reflection of your peer group's expectations. I made a decision then to share with my peer group the importance of writing a book, both to keep me accountable and because I want them to feel free to share their dreams with me so I can encourage them.

After a lunch break, we moved on to another speaker. He helped us identify the person we want to be. For me, it is a writer. He asked us to write a sixty-second pitch of what qualified us to make our dreams happen. My answers were: I innately have been able to write, and I've experienced a stroke and have learned so much during this journey that I want to share—I truly desire to help others and to share my knowledge and experiences.

He reminded us that we are what we are consuming, so cautioned us to really pay attention to whom we are talking, what we are watching on TV, and what we are reading. All these thoughts I found worth considering.

Oh, how I enjoyed the next speaker. He started his career

as a writer researching story writing. He identified that every good story has four characters—a victim, a villain, a hero, and a guide.

The *victim* makes the hero look good; he/she's a prop for the villain; has no good role in real life; and rarely transforms. When you play victim, you suck energy from others.

The *villain* makes the hero look good and strong; usually has a back story of pain and wants others to experience the same pain. The story is over when the villain "goes down."

The *hero* is what the story is about. He/she is tough; faces challenges; acts with courage and faith; runs to the glimmer of light; and transforms to a better version of themselves. Life usually ends up great or teaches a greater lesson.

The *guide* helps others; is often someone who is older and has the goal to share their wisdom.

All of these characters are options we have in life. I recognized that for the past year, I've spent more time than necessary in the victim role. I see that I've been a hero for a few and desire to be more of a guide. The speaker's recommendation was that we play the hero so we can become the guide. I love that thought.

We talked about grieving the loss of some activities. Instead of considering life around Covid quarantine, I considered life around cognitive impairments with my stroke. I've grieved the loss of travel; income and the freedom to spend money; the easy use of my computer; being in groups of people; and being able to carry on conversations—they are almost impossible once I've hit sudden and unpredictable mental fatigue.

The theme of this conference was courage; we talked about fear being a reaction and courage a decision. Courage isn't something you store up; it's something you use. Life shrinks or expands based on your courage. We identified leadership qualities we admire. I was pleased to read the list back and see those traits in myself. To my core, I heard the speaker as he said, "You are enough!" What a wonderful day I had listening to this information, these teachings. I came away feeling motivated and on the right path to move forward.

(About two hours after it was done I had one of the worst headaches I'd had in a long time. It lasted from Saturday evening to Monday afternoon. I also slept off and on for most the next two days. Still, I would say this conference was worth it. No regrets.)

## *May 4*

I have gained eight pounds since we started self-isolating on March 15. Today I commit to daily moving for thirty minutes, consciously upping my water intake, paying attention to my food intake, and putting more intention on getting a good night's sleep.

Saskatchewan has entered Phase One of re-opening the province. Blair and I agree that we will continue to stay home and stay safe for a while yet.

## *May 19*

An odd and worrying occurrence today: Blair left very early this morning to go to the city with a friend. Last night he set out some oatmeal so he could have a little something to eat before he left. We agreed that I might get up with him, but if I were sleeping well I would stay in bed for a sleep-in. As it happened, I heard him get up but was able to fall back to sleep, and I slept soundly for another hour or so. It was good to wake up to coffee already made. I lounged in my pajamas and savoured the quiet morning with my coffee.

At about 11:30, I thought I might fry a few eggs for lunch. When I went to the fridge I saw that we were out of eggs. Darn! There was some leftover bacon though, so I thought I'd fry it up. I warmed the frying pan and put the bacon in. Oh, I love the smell of bacon. When I went to the cupboard to grab a dish I noticed a carton of eggs sitting near the sink. I thought that was odd because Blair had said he would have oatmeal. I figured he must have decided to have eggs and forgot to put them away. So now, I figured, I can have eggs with my bacon. As I grab an egg from the carton I'm surprised by how cold it is. I thought it would have been warmer, having already been on the counter for more than three hours.

Blair arrived home around 5 p.m., and we chatted about our day. For some reason, I remembered that the eggs were left out and I asked him if he decided oatmeal wasn't enough this morning. He said he didn't have eggs. Just the oatmeal. And I really had to think about this. If he hadn't taken out the eggs, I must have. That would explain why they were cold.

I was very unsettled by having absolutely no memory of taking them out of the fridge. I didn't even have that "oh yeah—I kinda remember putting them on the counter" moment. Nothing! I remembered nothing!

This was a small moment, I realize, but this isn't the first time I've been made aware that I still have memory lapses.

I wonder what else I'm forgetting. I feel bad that my head goes to assuming Blair has done something off or wrong, when really it's me.

Here, on the cusp of the first anniversary of my stroke, I'm still finding inconsistencies from my pre-stroke life to that of my life today.

## *What I have learned ...*

**Do all you can to continue to learn and grow.** If you're unable to read, tune into motivational and/or educational webinars. If looking at monitors bothers your head, tune into podcasts and audio books. There is so much wisdom out there that can guide us to living the best life we can, brain injury or not, regardless of our circumstances.

**Acceptance of your post-brain injury abilities will help to protect your quality of life.** Dwelling, in a negative way, on limitations you now experience can become overwhelming. Push yourself to focus on what you *can* do and grow from there.

# PART TWO

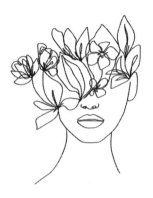

## Year Two – Quarter One

### *May 2020*

May 21 is both our 32$^{nd}$ wedding anniversary and the one-year anniversary of my stroke. Even with Covid, we receive anniversary deliveries of flowers and a special low-carb meal that Justine arranged through her friend's restaurant. And a lovely call from Jared. It was a wonderful day! We have so much to be grateful for—Blair is still with us and we get to celebrate another anniversary, and I've come a long way with my stroke recovery. I have improved balance and comprehension and am able to drive and read, even if only for short spurts.

One of my recent goals was to complete a 10-km walk. One day, a fun post shows up on my Facebook page encouraging people to do a virtual walk/run, called The Sloth Run. I think the name is hilarious and appropriate for the way I am feeling—kind of slow and sluggish. Participants in this walk/run are asked to donate to the Wildlife Federation, and they will receive a medal for their accomplishment. With daily walks of progressively longer stretches, I work my way up to be able to do the 10-km walk and complete it successfully by the end of May. This is a huge accomplishment. I am proud both of meeting a goal I had set, as well as being physically able to do the walk all on my own. (Instead of relying on touching my walking partner to recover from a feeling of imbalance, I was able to touch a building, or a fence, or a tree.) I celebrated the fact that there is still a lot out there for me to accomplish!

Throughout these Covid days, Mom continues to require a doctor's care, but we manage to handle this successfully, although there are plenty of Covid hoops to jump through. She loves the outings, even if it is just being in the car to her appointments and straight back home. Each appointment requires a two-week isolation in her room at the care home, but we are both starved for the hug and peck on the cheek we can have when we see each other, and that carries us for the intervening weeks. We have become good at visiting through her bedroom window or, on nice days, settling into our respective sides of the fence in her backyard.

I tried to push the limits of my independence by driving Mom to Moose Jaw to an appointment. It didn't go well. I have to sleep in the car to rest my brain before I am able to drive us safely back home. I spend the next day fighting a headache, brain fog, and fatigue. I'm not sure driving more than fifteen or twenty minutes is in the cards for me. For the safety of myself and others, I resign myself to not trying to drive any great distance unless I have another driver with me to take over.

I find that I am still learning my limits and, like a child, pushing the boundaries when I get frustrated and want to spread my wings a little more.

Post-stroke is still a journey. I forget that my brain is still healing. Having said that, I don't want to become complacent and assume there are tasks I simply can't do. I still need to try and find out for myself what limitations still exist. I play this game with myself: If there is something important that I want to accomplish, I tell myself that it is my "job" to work at it until it's completed. Some days that means getting up and dressing in my office clothes to keep myself in the right mindset. I keep my "work days" manageable, maybe one hour max at the computer screen. I'm still not accustomed to the slow pace but am grateful to be accomplishing tasks.

This process is especially effective when I decide that a good thing to do during our Covid stay-at-home is to paint all the walls (except in the bedrooms and bathroom) in our condo. My work outfit is my paint clothes, and I am "on the clock" for an hour and a half in the morning and the same in the afternoon. It takes a full week, but the walls look fresh and clean when I am done. I was very conscious of how just two small steps on the stepladder played havoc with my balance. In the end, it was another job completed!

## *June 2020*

My last official day as the Member Relations Officer at Southland Co-op is June 4, twelve and a half months after my stroke. I really enjoyed this job and all the staff I worked with. For months, I have worked at wrapping my head around being "retired" instead of "unable." I remain positive by celebrating the fact that I have this time to spend with Blair. I know that we will enjoy our time together and trust that the finances will work themselves out. I applied for CPP Disability in April 2020 but, as I have said, I understand that the processing takes more than four months in most cases. Knowing this, we set aside funds and prepaid bills. I did look into EI benefits but didn't qualify because I hadn't had 600 hours of employment in the past 52 weeks.

We've become very efficient at shopping when we are in the city. We prepare a short list and then we divide and conquer. I suspect, but am not sure, that I may be more tolerant of the visual and audio stimulation in most stores if I go in highly focused; it may help me to block out some of the external "noise."

We are told that Blair's cancer is active again in several lymph nodes around his trachea, stomach, and right lung. It is like someone pulled the power cord on my brain. I just had to sleep. Depression? Maybe. Does emotional stress cause mental fatigue? Maybe.

We have several medical appointments in a few weeks' span. Blair has a scan on his brain since the chemo he currently is on doesn't cross the blood-brain barrier, so his brain has been unprotected. After the scan, the oncologist changes the medication. We are feeling numb. We have been down this road before and Blair has conquered every challenge. *Lord, give him the strength to do it again. Amen.* Faith does not mean trusting God to stop the storm but trusting Him to strengthen us as we walk through the storm.

Within the week, we receive the results of the scan; the report says that there is no evidence of metastatic disease.

We spend the remainder of June and early July camping, on Blair's "good days." A change of chemo medication takes his system some time to get used to. There's something so calming and good for the soul to be out in the fresh air, bare feet on the grass, cool nights around a campfire and visits with family and friends around a picnic table. Medicine for the soul.

## *July 2020*

In early July, an intense hailstorm hits our hometown and we have hail damage at our condo. I was dreading getting on the computer to put in the claim. Thankfully, I am able to get online and do the bare minimum to get the insurance ball rolling. I can't wrap my head around attaching pictures and hope the report from the hail adjuster coming to look at our home will be sufficient. Between Blair's health challenges and the hailstorm, I find I need to have lengthy naps during the day just to keep up.

By late July, we start seeing Covid cases in our community, so we have a renewed commitment to stay home and stay safe. Although we chose to self-quarantine, the warm summer weather allows us an opportunity to enjoy our balcony that much more. Neighbours walking by stop to chat, and the elderly man across the street parks his scooter close enough that we can enjoy short conversations.

Stitching projects fill my days. I need to limit myself to no more than an hour at a sitting, especially with a new pattern. Beyond that, my eyes struggle to focus and the headaches at night return with a vengeance. It seems that with any new task I need to start very slowly and work at gaining endurance.

During one five-day stretch, I experience headaches that were worse than normal. I also had fatigue, napping a lot during the day and then sleeping all night. My appetite is poor and I have nausea, blurred vision, and dizziness. Because Covid had been confirmed in our community, it seemed wise to arrange to have a Covid test. The results were negative, thankfully.

Oddly, my left hip and thigh are painful, like a toothache. My thoughts seem particularly sluggish. When talking with Blair, at times, I really have to work hard to find my words. Blair wonders if maybe I was having another stroke. But all these symptoms are familiar to me. In 2004, I had West Nile virus. With the hip and thigh pain, headaches, and extreme fatigue, I am reminded of what I went through back then.

Four days after the Covid test, my symptoms resolve, thankfully.

## *August 2020*

I have been hacked— twice! First my Netflix account, and now my email account. All of my inbox, outbox, junk, and trash files have been deleted, as well as all my contacts. In the meantime, the hacker has contacted almost everyone in my personal, work, and home business contact lists asking them to touch base with me because I need their help. The email responses were redirected to the hacker who posed as me, writing that I was out of town and asking the recipients to purchase three $100-iTune cards. Then they were asked to send the activation codes from the back of the iTunes cards so that I could send them to my niece as a birthday gift. Of course, the activation codes would go to the hacker. I am both humbled and terrified at the number of friends and relatives who contact me to help out. I'm grateful for their offers to help and that they thought to check with me first. I would feel terrible if anyone was out $300 because of this scam!

Oh, what a nightmare. It was all my head could do to get in and change passwords and ensure my banking information is protected.

I experience extreme mood swings. Possibly related to

my diet? I wonder. I feel more-than-usual frustration at having to work so hard at things that used to be so easy. I struggle to find an activity to self-soothe, since reading isn't an option and yoga classes still have not resumed. I don't walk much, with the warm weather and increase in mosquito activity. Determined to find something that will help with my mental health, I find my favorite author on the library app. I can enjoy listening to the book for about thirty minutes before mental fatigue kicks in. Walking while listening to the audio book is exactly what I needed.

Soaking in the tub with an audio book playing was (and still is) very soothing for me. I settle into the warm water as the narrator shares the story. I enjoy listening to the plot unfold and old, familiar characters being introduced with just enough background information to jog my memory of previous novels. I'm grateful again for the "high cognitive reserve" that has stored these memories away. What surprises me is the emotional memories. I think that is why I enjoy reading so much—I enjoy being so submersed in a story (and the tub!) that I can make an emotional connection. With every chapter that I listen to, I feel a small spark returning, like a corner of my soul has colour returning to it. Have I been living in fear and frustration so long that I've lost sight of passion, intrigue, joy, and the comfort of intellectual stimulation? I can listen for quite a while without a headache. Maybe because I have nodded off in the tub for a bit and rested my mind, or maybe because I'm healing and making progress.

I do have a problem sometimes with audio books. I will start listening at Chapter 2, then suddenly it's Chapter 4, then Chapter 7. One day it was Chapter 20 and then it felt that all too soon it was Chapter 27. Is the narrator missing announcing the chapters? Am I zoning out? Am I actually falling asleep? Am I experiencing memory losses? This isn't the first time I've questioned my memory lately.

I found something else that is good for my mental health—time with our grandpup. We dog-sat Justine's dog, Lexi, for a few days. It is such fun to see the personality of this furry little pooch shine through. For us, it is like having a small child back in the house—early mornings, toys strewn throughout the living room, loving kisses and cuddles, regular walks and play time, even moments of "attitude" when no one responds to her rolling the ball under the entertainment stand for the fourth time in an hour. She is such fun to have for a visit.

In mid-August, I follow up on my CPP Disability application that I submitted on April 17. Initially I was told it would take 105 days to process, which would have been August 6. When I made the follow-up call, I was told it's 180 days and to not expect a response before

October 20. Again, we review our finances and plan how we can stretch to the next goal date. Some delays are being blamed on Covid. I'm learning patience, that's for sure.

I thought I'd try something—maybe if I drive and listen to an audio book, I won't be so focused on the ditches that seem to move by me faster than the road. I haven't been able to get over that sensation. The day ends in a headache, though it is hard to say whether the experiment was the cause, or if it is from visiting with seven people after the drive. Still so much trial and error to find where there might be a "sweet spot" that will let me comfortably do what I want or need to do.

Sometimes I feel like I'm my own science experiment. I've been monitoring my sleep score, as reported on my smart watch, to see if listening to a sleep meditation makes a difference to my quality or quantity of sleep. My sleep score has been consistently higher on the nights I use the meditations. Even more interesting, my estimated oxygen variation is much lower on nights when I listen to the sleep meditation recordings. I awake feeling much more refreshed and positive.

Blair is having more good days than bad. We decide, after five months of Covid quarantine, that we will take our 30-year-old motorhome to Ontario. We could visit family from six feet away and stay in our self-isolation.

It is late August and I am having an incredibly irritable spell. Some days, I can't even stand myself. I know Blair is going through his own struggles and yet I find myself snapping at him. I feel almost angry that his cancer again threatens to take him from me. I have to remind myself it's not him, it's the cancer that is throwing out the threat. I feel like my filters aren't working as well as they used to. I am saying hurtful words to people I care about, words that used to be held safe inside my head and heart knowing that cooler times would prevail. Blair and I eventually have a moment of airing our frustrations, crying because we don't want to hurt each other but knowing that things need to change. We both need to change. Like a pressure cooker finally able to vent, we both feel better. Tears followed by hugs, some boundaries were set, and we feel solid in our relationship again and somehow cleansed.

I try not to focus on finances. We'd been able to pay our bills but not having a paycheque since June 8th had certainly made us very aware of our spending. So why did we take a risk with Covid to travel east? Why spend the money? Because I don't know that Blair will be well enough next summer to travel. Because I can't expect all my family to travel here to see him. Because my dad is 90 and I want to be near him, even if Covid prevents me from visiting him in his care centre. I just want him to know I'm close. I need my sister and brother to hug me. I need them to know they will have a good visit with Blair. I need to laugh like only they can make me laugh.

I continually remind myself that I still totally trust that God has a plan and a purpose for me. I know that spending more time with Blair is the true blessing in all this and I'll forever be grateful for that. God knows my heart. He knows I'm frustrated and incredibly angry and my response some days is less than Christian, and I cry and I stomp my feet and I pray for forgiveness and strength and, most of all, peace.

Some days, what brings me out of what feels like a very selfish and angry state of mind is a close couple who are our friends. He is in the treatment part of their cancer journey, and that reminds me that things could be so much worse for us, and that we are in a place where we can be grateful.

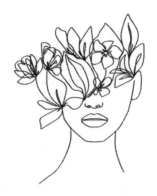

# Year Two – Quarter Two

## September 2020

From August 20 to September 11, 2020, we take a fabulous trip to Ontario in our home on wheels. We trust Bessie, our thirty-year-old motorhome, to get us to Ontario and back. Every day is an adventure, and we are grateful for each day of travel or visiting with family and friends.

While on the highway, I work with numbers and calculate our gas mileage and record expenses. I find it helps my brain to keep practising with numbers and it is pretty easy to do the calculations after a few days.

For the most part, my head handles this adventure well. I find conversations with more than a few people tiring. One day I went shopping with my sister, but I found it overwhelmed my head. I had to sleep during the short trip back home and then again once we got to her house. I still get excited for things that have been fun in the past. There are times I don't think about or anticipate how tiring a shopping trip will be. I just go. There are also times I consider the consequences but decide the outing is worth it. Often, my mental fatigue is delayed. Fortunately, this means that my evening sleeps are very restful.

During our travels, we stay in the motorhome in our families' yards. We eat meals with them but sleep in our own space to stay as self-contained and safe as possible. The only exception to this was when I spent four nights at my sister's house. She planned a Girls' Night at an Escape Room Adventure place with our nieces and our niece's friend. I love the mental challenge of these escape rooms. It is fun to be with the girls and I appreciated how quickly they were able to solve the puzzles.

During a family supper with Blair's cousin, his cousin asks those of us around the table what is on our bucket list. I am surprised how this hits me—I begin crying. For seven years, I've done my very best to be sure there was nothing left on Blair's bucket list. I think what was so emotional for me was that I hadn't thought about my own bucket list for years. Once I compose myself, I share that my wish is to go on a European riverboat cruise with my sister to visit Budapest, as our family roots go back to Hungary.

After we arrive home, I spend time again pondering my bucket list. I realize this may sound a bit commonplace for a bucket list, but what I do want to be able to do in my lifetime is to successfully make a piecrust! My cousin had made several pies effortlessly while we were visiting. She was gracious enough to give me a pie-making tutorial. I wrote many notes. To give a bit of background—when Blair and I were first married, I tried many times to make a good piecrust and whole wheat bread. I was able to master the bread but never the piecrust. That was always a thorn in my side. It has become a new short-term goal to try again! I feel surprisingly anxious just getting started. Once I have everything prepared and am ready to get my hands in the dough, I feel more confident that I can do it. Although it wasn't the most attractive pie, it was a peach pie that I knew Blair would enjoy. Even before it is done baking, I feel the mental fatigue come on. I cancel my plans for the rest of the day.

Within a few days of my first attempt at a piecrust, I stubbornly try to improve on my technique and to put out a better-looking pie. Just as I finish, a friend messages me and asks if I want to play a few hands of canasta. I really enjoy playing cards and think I'll go and hope that the post-pie fatigue won't hit.

I am able to stay awake but still feel a little emotionally raw. I know this may sound like an exaggeration but not being able to make a piecrust worth eating was one of those things that made me feel unaccomplished and inept. Funny how just making a piecrust brought back those insecurities. As we play cards and my friend teases me about little things, I find that I am super-sensitive. It feels like her words keep beating me down (that is my interpretation, and not her intent). It is probably a combination of feeling hurt by the words and the anxiety from the pie-making, and I am in an awkward space where I feel I want to leave before I start crying. I ask myself: Where is this coming from? Why now? Am I just overtired from our travel? I know my friend is caring and would never intentionally be hurtful. I come home and sleep, twice.

I continue to feel frustrated, as these emotional responses are still so unpredictable.

I am having muscle cramps in my neck. They start on the left side near my endarterectomy scar and sometimes are so severe that they turn my head. I am also experiencing heartburn but wonder if it is connected to something I have eaten. The frequency of the neck cramping increases over a two-week period. I call the doctor's office but can't book a phone consult for a week. I am concerned enough that I go to the ER. An ECG is completed, and blood work is taken. No heart concerns although my blood pressure is 178/104 and the upper number stays in the 170s for three hours. I am given a medication and prescription to help with the heartburn. I think maybe this is an anxiety-related problem, since heart concerns were ruled out. Another reminder to plan more self-care.

## *October 2020*

In mid-October, I feel generally overwhelmed with the unknowns of the future and financial uncertainty. Still no word from CPP Disability. We are doing remarkably well in meeting our financial responsibilities. Although I know all the things to do to stay positive and to support my mental health, I am struggling. Our insurance doesn't cover the cost of a counsellor, which would have been ideal. I commit to following what I have learned so far on my journey so I can get back to a more positive state of mind.

By late October, I was once again in touch with CPP. I was asked, kindly, if I thought I could work at any type of job. I really had to give this some thought. After a few days of sincere contemplation, I sent this response to the CPP office:

## *Am I able to go back to any type of job?*

- *Multi-tasking overwhelms my brain sometimes. I think maybe I could pump gas, which would be fine if there were only one vehicle. If a second vehicle pulled up and asked for gas and asked me to check the oil or, heaven forbid, a third vehicle pulled up, I know I'd be mentally overwhelmed. At home if I'm following a recipe, the phone rings, and hubby asks me a question all at once, that's enough to bring on a wave of extreme fatigue. If I hold my hand up in a "stop" sign motion or say "too much," my husband knows I'm struggling and steps up to help. Can I do that at a job? Will my employer tolerate sudden, unpredictable needs for me to nap 20 minutes, or, on some days, to nap frequently for an entire afternoon?*

- *Could I do an office job? I try to do tasks on my laptop at home to keep my skills up and check my screen-time tolerance. Some days I do pretty well for up to an hour. Some days I can't figure out how to print a document when I know I've done it mindlessly thousands of times in the past. Sometimes I'm extremely stubborn and stay with it, trying to figure it out to the point that my head aches and I am frustrated to tears. Some days I'm strong enough to walk away and not let it ruin my day. How do I fit this into a workday?*

- *Conversations are particularly tiring for me. I asked the psychologist about that. She explained that our brain is like an hourglass—the wide top takes in input, the narrowing is the area of processing, and the larger bottom is output. She said when too much is coming in (for me, conversations, large groups, being in a store, extreme emotional situations, etc.) it gets stuck in the "processing" bottleneck and my brain has to shut down to reset. That explains the "why"— but how do I fit that into a job/employment?*

- *I've been working in and around our community for over thirty years. I'm known as an upbeat, multi-tasking, community-minded extrovert. Where I worked most recently, my coworkers and my employers saw that I was unable to return to work and kindly spread the word that I "retired." I miss being part of the team. I miss getting up and getting dressed for work, I miss being the problem solver and the ideas person. Would I find a job and get back to it if I could? In a heartbeat!! Would I take a job and know that I would fail at it? Replace my reputation as an extremely good worker to a person who can't put in even a half day? My worry is not that the people who know me would judge me or be upset with me; it's more that they would pity the person I am now compared to who I was. And for what? Could I work three half-days a week? At minimum wage?*

*Would added stress, headaches, and losing the remainder of my days to fatigue really be worth the small income that will certainly help pay the bill, but barely?*

- *My husband has stage IV lung cancer. I have been his caregiver and now he's become mine. He absolutely thinks that my trying to find a job is a bad idea. He knows what life is like just here at home when tasks of daily living are too much. Is it fair of me to fight to get back to work and know that my quality of life and the consequences of working are going to affect him daily as well?*

- *I've owned two businesses over the years. I put myself in the employer's shoes. Training is expensive.*

- *I tried to learn how to bake a piecrust and, within the hour, extreme fatigue set in and lasted all day. Even with three to four afternoon naps I couldn't function. The way that tired me mentally, I would not have been able to drive home if I had to.*

- *Would I hire me? Based on work history and reputations, yes. Based on skills I currently have to offer, I'm not sure I'd make it past a probationary period. I'd be embarrassed to have the same frustrated meltdowns and the extreme fatigue episodes at someone's place of employment that I am challenged with frequently here at home.*

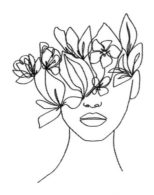

# Year Two – Quarter Three

## *November 2020*

As we approach the Christmas season in the comfort and safety of our home, we start decorating early and put up our tree the last week of November. We settle into a nesting frame of mind. I'm feeling safe and comfortable. I figure out how to listen to audio books on our Echo device. As part of my self-care, I stitch the tree topper and ornaments for our tree from plastic canvas. (I received some sage advice early on in this journey that things like puzzling, handwork, and even playing cards keeps your mind in the present and not worrying about the future. This seems to be the key for me.) The cooler winter weather brings on Blair's and my tradition of sharing a pot of tea, a very comforting way to end our day.

It is late November and I go to the optometrist to see if there is anything that can be done with my glasses to reduce the number of headaches I am experiencing. She referred me to an ophthalmologist. In the end, I am told that the issue isn't my eyes; it is my brain. This is not the news I'd hoped for, but now I know and I will continue to monitor my activities to do my best to keep headaches to a minimum.

The final approval for CPP Disability coverage is finally made! And back pay is granted. In the CPP Disability application, I signed the papers to have my group insurance company reimbursed for the months they paid me benefits when CPP Disability should have been my source of income. The regular monthly payments start in December 2020 and will continue until age 65 unless I have a return to health sufficient enough to be able to return to work.

I continue to listen and learn from podcasts. I firmly believe that I was meant to live a fulfilling, purposeful life. Sometimes I feel like the key to unlocking the wisdom of finding and living my purpose is just one idea, one concept away. During this time of searching, I listen to a particularly inspiring podcast. One of the things the speaker talks about is setting life goals. I like the idea of creating life goals and, as the speaker suggests, make it easy to remember by using an acronym to build on. I've decided my acronym would be VALUE:

**V** – **Value** life (maintain an aversion to the victim mindset).

**A** – Have an **attitude** of gratitude. In all things, find something to be grateful for. Some days, "fake it till you make it"— even if it's forced, find something to be grateful for.

**L** – Have faith, hope, and **love**—with the greatest of these being Love. I sincerely want to live each day having God's love shine through me. My prayer often is, *Lord, make me your instrument.*

**U** – **Unleash** my unknown potential. I'm totally trusting that God has a plan and a purpose for me in this life and I will remain open to whatever He has in store. Be open, observant, honest, and willing to step out in faith!

**E** – **Elevate**, **educate** and **empower** myself and others.

## *December 2020*

Most years in December, I make a vision board. This year, I joined a Zoom group to work on my vision board. I really enjoyed the afternoon of being inspired and joining in on the enthusiasm of the other participants. It was exciting to dream and envision my future—and, after three hours of screen time, I found my headache tolerable.

By mid-December, I am again ready to test my limits with driving. I drive half an hour in daylight and one hour at night, in darkness. I find the evening driving much easier, maybe because there are fewer visual distractions. Both times I have a passenger who is helping watch for wildlife. The ditch seems to move more in line with the speed of the road than it did in the months following my stroke, likely because my passenger provides the extra watching that I needed.

I am stitching some projects for Christmas gifts. Sometimes I push beyond what feels comfortable just to finish a piece—never to the point of visual disturbances though. I've learned that the barrier is there to help me and not something to be broken through. I feel like I have a better sense of what will happen if I push too hard.

I find that when I do too much stitching or have too much screen time, the following morning my eyes are almost tender—almost like tender muscles after a long walk or a workout that remind me in my first few movements of what I've done the day before.

I continue to have random anger outbursts. Unfortunately, with our attempts to "stay home, stay safe" it means that Blair is taking the brunt of these. I surprise even myself with how creative I am with finding something to be angry about, just to let off this spout of angry steam. It reminds me of the days when I had hormonal flares on blue days or teary days. Even then I didn't know what I was blue about or why I felt a need to cry; I just wanted it to pass, as I knew it would.

I'm finding that my filters still aren't totally intact, and I am still speaking my mind more than I used to. I kid myself that this may not be so much the result of the stroke as a convenient time to make a change to my response to being treated unfairly or unkindly. It was embarrassing at first for me but now feels quite liberating.

I sleep well 80 percent of the time. I wake up feeling more energized and ready to complete my goals for the day. I think that before my CPP disability was approved, I was continuing to push myself to spend time on the laptop and relearn some skills that I felt I'd lost. I'm spending less time doing this now and headaches, especially during the night, have decreased.

Reading for short periods of time (fifteen to twenty minutes) is now comfortable, both hardcopy books, and on a computer screen. Afterward, I have no headaches and my comprehension remains good. Listening to audio books and podcasts keeps my mind satisfied and I enjoy being able to still learn. I realize that it was reading on a computer screen, not just looking at the screen, that had been difficult.

Being in stores still makes my head spin. Walking alone is much easier now. My balance is better. Only rarely do I find the movement in my peripheral vision distracting enough to make me feel unsteady. Too much conversation still seems to tire my brain. We haven't been in large groups for months so I am not sure how that would feel now.

Being in highly emotional situations feels like the power cord of my brain has been jerked out of the socket. Strong feelings of fear, anger and sadness seem to be the worse. I need to sleep, sometimes for only a few minutes and sometimes up to half an hour, to "recharge." On a really emotional day, recharging naps throughout the day seem to be the only way I can function.

The most calming times for me are stitching, puzzling,

cooking, or baking. I continue to have regular one-on-one coffee dates with friends. We keep these under an hour and they are very enjoyable.

I play canasta about three or four times a month. That feels like a good brain exercise. I often have a headache the night of the game, but it's one of those things I enjoy enough to put up with the discomfort.

At almost nineteen months post-stroke, I'm feeling more content, maybe because I've quit trying so hard to "get better." I am enjoying more what I can do rather than worrying about when I'll get back to what I used to do.

I am continually grateful for my "high cognitive reserve" that continues to give me confidence. There are still days when I have random thoughts about some technical information that isn't necessarily helpful at the time but gives me a sense of confidence that there is still knowledge stored away that will be there when I need it one day.

Just before Christmas, during my morning gratitude practice, I realize that I have finally shed the victim role. I am not sure exactly when or why that happened; I just know that once I recognized I was wearing that role, I realized how heavy it had become—a not-so-silent burden. I am relieved to have it gone. Happy to be happy again.

Christmas, for the most part, is cancelled this year due to Covid. I have to admit that although this change has been different, it hasn't been all bad. We have time to make homemade gifts, send Christmas cards (haven't done that in a decade), cook the turkey and cabbage rolls early, and make Christmas care packages. Video chats are booked for Christmas Day.

I had an interesting online chat with a friend. As another year was coming to an end, there was excitement in thinking about what the new year will bring. We talked about goals and desires for what our lives could/should look like. We wondered about desires—do we have desires first and then pray that God will work in our lives to make them happen, or does God put the desires on our heart as a precursor to a blessing? Sometimes praying for things we desire seems too selfish or greedy so we are hesitant to go down that path. We talked about things I had on my vision board—the greatest being the writing and publishing of my book. I feel like it's meant to be, but I have no idea how to work through the editing and publishing process. I booked a visit with a friend who has self-published a book, and prepared lots of questions for her. If my book is meant to be out there to help others, I totally trust that God will prepare the path.

As December comes to an end, I spend more time writing. I try to pace myself and do little bits each day, but that has evolved into one-hour stretches once or twice a day. My headaches have returned with a vengeance and my vision is really poor by the afternoon. I take a break from writing until everything settles down, and then I am able to get back to it.

## *January 2021*

New year, new beginnings. Writing is replaced with puzzling for a time. I want to increase my stamina by pushing the limits with my vision. Even though I am uncomfortable, I am enjoying the mindless challenge of finding another piece.

I started a personal growth 21-day challenge on January 1, 2021. I am very introspective. I enjoy self-growth opportunities, especially when they can be done all online at my own pace. It gives purpose to getting up and starting the day—it is my "job." It adds intention for the day, as each day there is an action plan that sometimes is as simple as journaling some of my past challenges, consciously choosing not to participate in negative conversations, or paying attention to my negative thoughts and turning them into positive thoughts. Surprising how this changes my day for the better.

Sadly, our motorhome had been written off—due to rodent infestation! We are very excited to have found a camper to replace it. We are thrilled to find one with everything we had on our wish list—the list I had noted on my vision board less than a month ago. Even better, the seller has agreed to let us make four payments so we can pay it off in April and be ready for the camping season. Life feels exciting!

Early in January, I listen to the following story online and realize I have had a tainted perspective of how my life has been since the stroke. I see now that I was exactly where I'd always wanted to be—spending time with Blair.

*One day a fisherman was lying on a beautiful beach, with his fishing pole propped up in the sand and his solitary line cast out into the sparkling blue surf. He was enjoying the warmth of the afternoon sun and the prospect of catching a fish.*

*About that time, a businessman came walking down the beach, trying to relieve some of the stress of his workday. He noticed the fisherman sitting on the beach and decided to find out why this fisherman was fishing instead of working harder to make a living for himself and his family.*

*"You aren't going to catch many fish that way," said the businessman to the fisherman.*

*"You should be working rather than lying on the beach!"*

*The fisherman looked up at the businessman, smiled and replied, "And what will my reward be?"*

*"Well, you can get bigger nets and catch more fish!" was the businessman's answer.*

*"And then what will my reward be?" asked the fisherman, still smiling.*

*The businessman replied, "You will make money and you'll be able to buy a boat, which will then result in larger catches of fish!"*

*"And then what will my reward be?" asked the fisherman again.*

*The businessman was beginning to get a little irritated with the fisherman's questions. "You can buy a bigger boat and hire some people to work for you!" he said.*

*"And then what will my reward be?" repeated the fisherman.*

*The businessman was getting angry. "Don't you understand? You can build up a fleet of fishing boats, sail all over the world, and let all your employees catch fish for you!"*

*Once again, the fisherman asked, "And then what will my reward be?"*

*The businessman was red with rage and shouted at the fisherman,*

*"Don't you understand that you can become so rich that you will never have to work for your living again! You can spend all the rest of your days sitting on this beach, looking at the sunset. You won't have a care in the world!"*

*The fisherman, still smiling, looked up and said, "And what do you think I'm doing right now?"*

I continue to enjoy outings with friends. During a coffee I had with a fellow massage therapist, our conversation came around to my book. I shared with her my new vision for the book. I shared my struggles with her. Is pursuing my goal to write a book an ego trip? My true heart's desire is to help others. She said she saw the massage therapist in me that always provided education for aftercare for my clients. I loved that! Early after my stroke I just wanted someone to step up and lead me through my recovery as I had done with so many massage clients. The book, I thought, would allow me to fulfill that therapeutic step for others on the same post-traumatic head-injury journey.

I enjoy listening to Mathew McConaughey's *Greenlights* audio book. He speaks of paths that were meant for him to travel. When he realizes he's exactly where he was meant to be, he says "Green Light." This makes me think of my own "Green Lights":

I'm spending my days with Blair as he enjoys "good days." – Green Light

I'm preparing a book so I can help others on this same journey. – Green Light

I've rediscovered the creative side of me as I stitch projects and Christmas decorations. – Green Light

I'm enjoying in-person and video coffee dates with more and more friends. My personal relationships are blossoming. – Green Light

I am enjoying self-help podcasts and books that I'm able to listen to daily. My craving for new information has been satisfied. My curious self is fulfilled. – Green Light

I'd made it a priority to move thirty minutes each day, and am feeling healthier, sleeping better. – Green Light

This past summer we had a great adventure when we drove out to Ontario to visit family and friends. We didn't need to rush back. Enjoyed the leisurely pace, the beautiful scenery, lots of time outside and all the visits. Enjoyed strengthening bonds and creating memories with Blair. – Green Light

## *February 2021*

I have found a new experience I am curious to know if I can master. I am both excited and a little terrified to try out my first spin class in Rockglen 50 kms away. Justine has given me tips on how to make it to the end of the class and encouraged me to only do what was comfortable for this first class and then next class push a little more. It is good to see familiar faces at the class as well as another first-timer. Everyone is encouraging and helpful. I hadn't really thought about it but the bike I am riding is right beside the speaker. In the past, loud noises brought on an imbalance in my gait and brain fatigue. The music is upbeat and I know the songs, so focusing on the beat and lyrics is a great distraction to the dizzy way my head is starting to feel. I manage pretty well.

When it is time to approach the standing position I realize that standing is not a good decision. I feel incredibly off balance. I give myself permission to be happy with completing the class without stopping even if I remain seated the whole time. The instructor remains upbeat as she says, "Now grab your weights and we'll sit upright while pedaling and do a little work with the weights." *Can I?* I wonder. Sitting up actually steadies my head and I feel a surge of energy. When I walk and start to feel dizzy, I know that ears over shoulders over hips will calm the sensation of imbalance. I consciously sit up and maintain the good postural alignment. I made it through the weight portion of the class! I am so pleased to have maintained the rhythm of my feet spinning while performing the different weight exercises. I've got this!

Hands back on the handlebars. Oh darn, the dizziness had returned. My goal remains to make it to the end of the class. I did it! My head was spinning and I could feel the pressure of the headache but I did it! I was so tired. So grateful that Blair was willing and able to be my driver to and from Rockglen. (It was good to be able to sleep 25 minutes of the 30-minute ride home.)

By the time we arrive home, the headache has built to a substantial level of discomfort so I jump in the tub for a soak in the hope of preventing too much muscle pain tomorrow and to soak off the sweat from the class. Would I do another class? Probably not any time soon. Am I pleased that I tried it and continued pedaling from start to finish? Yes, I am thrilled! I learned a lot and reinforced some of what I already knew. 1) I'm not afraid to try. 2) Posture is critical to help me feel balanced again when I get dizzy. 3) Loud sounds still have an effect on me, for now.

I have a great community of supporters that I am incredibly grateful for.

Although taking on this challenge terrified me, it feels like the old me is back. The younger, healthier version of me who was open to new experiences. Learning about myself and new opportunities. My curiosity has been quenched.

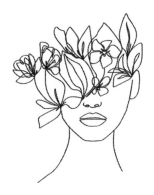

# Year Two – Quarter Four

## *March 2021*

At the end of my first year following the stroke, some professionals told me that the abilities I had at that point would be the abilities I'd be left with post-stroke. Some professionals said two years. As I near the second-year anniversary of my stroke, I have to admit that there hasn't been much change since my first-year anniversary, at least not cognitively. What I have noticed is the increase in peace, the reduced resistance to staying home, the increased appreciation of the opportunity to retire early, a commitment to write what I'm grateful for daily, and the renewed joy in my life.

Wednesday group video chats with Dad have become a part of my family's routine. Instead of the activity worker at his facility initiating the calls, my sister is able to go in and do it. Even with Covid restrictions, she is considered his Essential Visitor, and has been able to be with Dad three days a week. This video call in early April is unusual. My niece and I are telling Dad how handsome he looks with his new haircut. He looks like he is going to cry, and then it appears as though he was falling asleep. I ask if he wants to rest. He confirms that he does and we cut the call short. I call my sister later to see if Dad is okay, and she says it wasn't one of his better days. I feel worry in the pit of my stomach, concerned that something isn't right.

A few days later, Blair and I receive our first Covid vaccination. With his cancer and my stroke, we are considered high risk, so we both thought it was a good idea to have an extra level of protection. Psychologically, it is comforting to know we are doing all we can to stay safe and keep others safe too.

## *April 2021*

On April 10, we receive a call from my sister, who tells us that Dad has been admitted to hospital and is not doing well. She suggests that we might want to plan a trip to come home.

A prairie blizzard is on its way and we don't want to chance pulling our new-to-us camper through a winter storm with the new-to-us truck that has only been used for a local hunting trip a few months previously. By April 14th, roads are clear enough for us to finally head out for Ontario. Thankfully, Dad has remained stable. Within a few days, we have crossed the Ontario border and our fourteen-day Covid isolation countdown begins. By April 17th, we arrived at my brother's acreage and set up camp in his driveway.

We knew that, due to Covid, we were not able to go into the long-term care facility to see Dad unless "end of life was imminent." We understood the restriction and trusted that Dad would remain in reasonably good health, and I optimistically hoped we could continue with video visits. I was also hoping that Dad would take comfort in knowing that Blair and I, and my younger brother, had arrived safely from Saskatchewan and were near if he needed us.

Not a week had passed since our arrival when we were told we were able to go in to see Dad. I could hardly wrap my heart and mind around what that meant. Was he already in the "death is imminent" stage? I was both excited and anxious to go in and see him.

Our reunion was bittersweet. We were required to put

247

on mask and gown before entering his room. Oh how I hoped he would know it was me. Selfishly, I was glad we weren't required to wear gloves. I wanted the skin-to-skin contact of holding his hand. The nurse quietly gave me permission to take my mask down to give him a kiss—such a compassionate gesture on her part. I was so glad she was sensitive enough to allow us to share the tenderness of a kiss. Dad reached out to give Blair a firm, familiar handshake—his usual way of greeting friends and strangers alike.

As I sat at his bedside holding his hand, I was acutely aware of how soft it was. I remembered the weathered, calloused hands from my younger years when Dad spent his days farming the land, milking the cows, and working on farm equipment he'd sold to local farmers and ranchers.

I had left Ontario when I was 17. For the last nearly three-quarters of my life, I had been 1500 kilometres away from him. Now all of a sudden, I felt like I had missed so much. Dad interrupted my thoughts by telling me how glad he was that we were there and then, quietly but confidently said, "It's okay, I'm okay." I fought tears as I sensed that he was telling me he was ready to go home to his Lord.

The chaplain had been in to pray with Dad and play him

old hymns and songs he knew Dad would enjoy. Family members took turns going in to visit. It was a few days before Blair and I would go in again. By then, Dad was non-responsive, and each breath was a struggle. I had loved this man all of my life. I'd always felt comfortable coming home to visit and was always made to feel loved and appreciated. As I sat holding Dad's hand and listening to his laboured breathing, I found myself being so grateful that we were able to connect with our weekly video chats over the past few months. Dad's face always lit up as our images came on screen. He wasn't always able to keep up with the conversation, but you could tell he was just happy to be part of it. Without Covid, without a reason to set up these video calls, these last months with him would have only been an occasional phone call, with few words spoken before he'd say goodbye because his own stroke had made speech hard.

On April 28, Dad passed away.

The care facility invited us to be present as Dad's body was wheeled out of the building, and the staff had an opportunity to pay their respects as he left. We appreciated their invitation and were glad to be able to be there. He was draped in a beautiful quilt with the words "A life well lived" stitched at one end. Without a doubt, Dad had lived a good life. He had served his community. He had raised five children who were all hard-working, responsible adults he was proud of. He adored his grandchildren and great-grandchildren. His quiver was full.

The chaplain said a few kind words and a hymn was played. For the first time in these past, rushed days of driving to get there as quickly as possible, arriving and heading to the hospital sooner than we anticipated, it felt real. Dad was gone. Forever.

His funeral, in Covid times, was small. Immediate family only. The local funeral home that handled the funeral told us that some families share the details of when the family would leave the funeral home and when they were expected to arrive at the cemetery. Anyone who might want to pay their respects could park along the way as we drove Dad to his final resting place. So many friends and family lined the side of the highway. The most beautiful honour guard. We were all so touched by their effort to say goodbye to a kind, honourable man.

For days I was numb. I wanted to help my sister and brother with all the meetings and paperwork required to close the estate. It was so hard to keep my head in the game. I knew being too emotional would quickly tire my brain, and it did.

Within a few weeks we were back home in Saskatchewan. In fact, we arrived home one day after our 33rd wedding anniversary and the second anniversary of my stroke.

My peace had faded. My heart was aching. I decided then that I would allow myself time to grieve. After all, I had all the knowledge I had gathered to help get me back to a place of strength and peace once my mourning had subsided.

I acknowledged that Dad had taught me about hard work. About problem solving. About serving others. About being kind and honourable. I realized that these were all tools I had needed to climb over and through all the obstacles the stroke had laid in my path.

I knew Dad would be proud of how I had worked to stay positive and look for solutions to make life good again. I knew he'd be happy to see that I'd use this experience to help others.

From the heavenlies, I could almost feel him share the quote, "You've been assigned this mountain to show others it can be moved."

Thanks for all you've taught me, Dad; I will accept this challenge.

# PART THREE

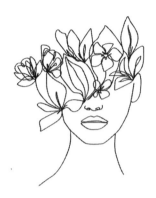

## Stepping Into the Future

As I complete the writing of this book, I'm happy to write that I'm in a space of greater joy and peace.

*What have I learned through this experience that I really want to share to help others?*

**Acknowledge emotion:** It is very common to experience anger and frustration following the event that damaged the brain. This could be caused by injury to the parts of the brain that control emotional expression. It could also be due to frustration and dissatisfaction with changes in life brought on by the injury (loss of job, physical abilities, and independence). Some people struggle with being isolated, depressed and/or misunderstood.

**Acceptance** of my new life and limitations was the starting point to embracing the new me. Different can be good. I find that being perfectly imperfect is far less stressful. Previously, I was so goal oriented that I lived life always on a mission. If I passed you on the street, I would politely say, "Hi" but my head was busy focusing on the goal I was trying to accomplish and that was where my thoughts were focused. Now, holding onto a thought or a goal is often fleeting. This frees my mind to welcome conversations with family and friends. I feel much more connected within my circle now. I love this part of the new me.

Another part of acceptance was giving myself permission to let go of the old me. I had to replace the anger of "I can'ts" with celebrating the "I can's" and be excited about discovering the new me. I had to affirm to myself that I wasn't giving up, I was letting go of the things I couldn't change. I regularly take stock of how far I've come, express gratitude for these successes, and acknowledge that I am perfectly imperfect and that's okay.

**Gratitude** is HUGE. Although it felt so fake at first, I really did have to "Fake it till you make it." Once I recognized that I was dwelling in a space of victimhood, one of the small steps I took to crawl out was finding things I could be grateful for. Initially small items of gratitude like having a warm blanket, the feeling of freshly brushed teeth and being able to figure out the TV remote began to evolve into more significant moments of appreciation. Grateful to have Blair's support, grateful to have found audio books and other educational audio resources, grateful to have very little residual physical impairments, grateful to relearn tasks even if the learning is temporary.

**Sleep** is incredibly important. I want to get the best sleep at night that I can. Also, when I have times of extreme fatigue due to too many mental challenges or exceptionally emotional events, it is important that I nap (whether it is for 20 minutes or 2 hours). I'll wake up when my brain is ready to go again. I've also learned to educate people in my social circle that there is the possibility that I will need to "rest." We can then make accommodations for a quiet space, if needed. Being able to comfortably set up some boundaries took a while for me, but became easier as people become more aware of my needs.

**Asking for help** is becoming so much easier. I think being uncomfortable in this area in the past had a lot to do with my ego. I would define ego, in this instance, as the part of "self" that is tied to my occupation, my educational background, my financial status and my abilities. When these are taken away you are stripped to the core of who "self" really is. Losing all those things was hard. I felt angry and lost for so long. I wanted "the old me" and my old life back. Once I accepted these parts of "me" were gone, I was pleasantly surprised to find that at the very core of "me" resides a caring woman that is energized by helping others. A woman I am proud of.

**Power to choose.** Event plus reaction equals outcome. It isn't always easy, but you have the power to choose how you respond to every life experience. You can choose your attitude. This has been the most valuable equation I've learned. When I get overwhelmed, I make my best effort to stand back, take a look at what's going on as though I was looking at someone else's life, and then choose how I'm going to react.

**Faith.** Throughout this experience my faith has remained strong. I believe with all my heart and mind that God loves me more than I can comprehend. I honestly believe that everything that has happened in my life has happened for me and not to me. Even through the months of anger and frustration, I remained curious about God's purpose in this experience. I see the blessings now. I've been given more time at home with Blair, watched my relationships with family and friends grow, I've found new ways to keep my inquisitive mind satisfied—I've even enjoyed walking more. Maybe it's this faith that gives me hope that my new life will be exactly what it's meant to be.

**Gratitude:** My wish is that sharing my story and struggles will help to encourage others finding their way through the experience of a new brain injury and ultimately provide hope that life can be better. In my case, I went from a terrifying stroke to a life of gratitude, hope, and grace.

# PART FOUR

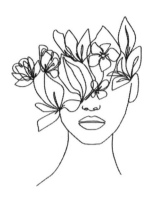

## Things to Know About Someone with a Brain Injury -
### ... And How You Can Help

1. We may still be trying to find our way back to the "old me" and are in a state of anger and frustration. You can help by listening and not trying to fix us. Especially early on when the anger and frustration is all encompassing.

2. We may be hesitant to go out in public. One particular concern is our new lack of filters, speaking comments that normally would be held private, resulting in embarrassment and regret. The weight of guilt from what we've inadvertently said can be too heavy to carry. You can help by planning small one-on-one visits. Let the conversations flow and understand the

comments come from a different place. Not from a space of judgement or criticism, but from an injury we had no control over.

3.   Memory loss is frightening. We may not remember a previous conversation or plans made. So much so, that we become defensive if we don't remember participating in the discussion or decision making. You can help by being flexible. Please don't tell us "Remember…." If we could remember, we wouldn't be arguing with you.

4.   Sudden rage is a thing. We're not always sure what brings it on. We may not even recognize we're in it until it passes. We likely are regretful when it passes. You can help by knowing the rage isn't about you or aimed at you.

5.   We miss our independence and ability to initiate adventure. You can help by creating an adventure, or experience … maybe a quiet drive to a new location or to discover a local historical site that you've driven by but never stopped to explore. Maybe an afternoon of fishing at a nearby lake, river or pond. If the adventure you're planning isn't local, pack a pillow and blanket for the drive and offer permission to rest as needed—or to do what we can together and allow the opportunity to comfortably say "I've had

enough." A modified adventure is still an adventure and can end with plans for the next experience.

6. We very likely regret that we've added worries and extra work to the lives of our friends and family members. You can help by assuring us that we are all learning together and remind us that this experience is new to you, too.

7. As much as we may grieve the loss of a loved one, we experience grief for the loss of our skills and abilities. You can help by brainstorming alternatives with us such as an audio book app for those who can no longer read, or a new hobby to help keep our hands and mind busy when we aren't able to return to work or to comfortably look at a computer screen any longer.

8. Financial struggles are compounded when you struggle with the cognitive capacity to work through solutions. When the brain injury is new and your income is suddenly in jeopardy, there is a huge adjustment to living within your new limited financial resources. You can help by offering some cost-effective solutions. You can offer to do the grocery shopping (remember stores are loud and visually over stimulating so shopping is a gift in and of itself). Cooking at home is a quick and easy

solution to reducing the outflow of cash. Maybe you could teach your friend how to cook your favorite dish, or spend some time together making freezer meals that can be easily put together and prepared for a healthy and satisfying meal, or, if you're in a good financial position, maybe pay for groceries and take that one expense off your friend's plate.

9.  We may experience sudden fatigue when emotions are high. Any emotion—fear, excitement, worry, anxiety, joy, anger—can affect us this way. You can help by being sensitive to this. When possible, calm down the situation that is evoking the emotions.

10. Our minds are usually sharpest and most alert and ready for mental challenges in the morning. You can help by taking advantage of our mornings for visits, for arranging this time for events that require decisions to be made or tasks to be performed.

11. From the faith-filled part of me, I truly believe that the greatest gift you can give us is to include us in your thoughts and prayers.

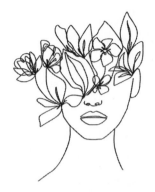

# What we would tell you
# if we could ...

- Neuro fatigue is a real thing, we aren't just lazy. If I say I am tired, I am REALLY tired.
- It's not always easy.
- Just because you can't see it, it doesn't mean it's not there. I may look alright but you have no idea what's going on inside of me and my brain.
- It takes time, please be patient. A new me is struggling to be born. Give her time and a chance.
- You kind of feel like a spirit – watching the world go by and go on without you.

- My brain isn't as slow as the rest of me. I am still able to think and reason.
- Sometimes I'm angry and impatient for no obvious reason. Please be patient and know it's not your fault. I know it's hard for you to understand. It's the same for me.
- My brain has a flip-phone battery in an iPhone world.
- We are not stupid; we are slow at processing information.
- Because I look okay, it doesn't mean I am okay.
- Life after our event may be different, but that does not mean it may not be worthwhile.
- It's hard to listen to people say you are not the same. And embarrassing when you say something that your brain doesn't process quick enough before your mouth said something stupid!
- We will figure out our new normal and then we figure out how to do things that way.
- It never goes away; it's always at the forefront of your mind, always second guessing, always wondering is this really me or my broken brain.
- Just thinking wears me out some days. To do two things at a time can exhaust me to the point of despair. I've never considered my brain and its function. I can no longer ignore my brain. My time doesn't flow like it used to.
- It is hell! I make so many mistakes. I hate it!

- If I tell you I can do something, I can. If I tell you I can't, I can't.
- I am not helpless, or stupid. I have a pretty good idea of my capabilities and my weaknesses. Trust me on that and let me do what I can.

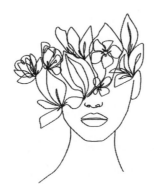

# Notes

## *Part One, Month One*

1   Jayaraj R.L., Azimullah S., Beiram R., Jalal F.Y., Rosenberg G.A. *Neuroinflammation: friend and foe for ischemic stroke.* Journal of Neuroinflammation. *2019;16(1):142*

2   *2019 Report on Heart, Stroke and Vascular Impairment.* Heart and Stroke Foundation of Canada. Taken from "(Dis)connected: How unseen links are putting us at risk."

3   *physiocanhelp.ca*

## *Part One, Month Two*

1   Taken in part from Brain Injury Society of Toronto article "Reducing screen time post ABI"

## *Part One, Month Three*

1   The Neuroscience of Gratitude and How It Affects Anxiety & Grief, *PositivePsychology.com,* Jan. 9, 2020

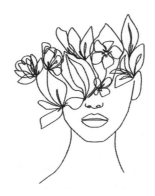

# Acknowledgements

I am grateful and thankful for you, Blair; my best friend, caregiver, cheerleader and love of my life. God has blessed me richly when he gifted me with you. Thank you for being my rock as we figure out what this new life after the stroke will look like. I admire your self-worth and compassion as you weather the storms of my unpredictable bouts of anger. Thank you for knowing that the anger was sometimes spewed at you but wasn't about you. As soon as it's done, we move on as though it had never happened even though I have regret that I've put you through it, again. I'm grateful that the season of anger is mostly behind us. Thank you for loving me when I struggled to love myself.  Thank you for always being supportive of the idea and intention of this book-to use my experience to help others. You encouraged me when the task of editing and publishing seemed insurmountable and when I questioned if my story was big enough and if I could really make a difference for someone else. I celebrate the completion of this book and every life that it will touch, with you.

Thank you, Jared and Justine, for making me the proudest mom. You both have worked through Dad and my health challenges with such grace. With all my heart I wish we could take back the worries we have created for you. Thank you for your support and encouragement after the stroke and with the writing of this book. Thank you for always being just a call or a text away.

Thank you, Mom, for being another great cheerleader. I know how frustrating it is for you to recognize your memory is failing. The fact that you remember to ask about the book and then celebrate its progress with me means more than I can put into words. You have always been an inspiration for me and a soft shoulder to lean on. You are a beautiful example of acceptance and choosing how we respond to what life has given us.

Dad, I miss you. I love the moments when I feel you near. Thank you for teaching us how to work hard, how to be honest and live with integrity. My prayer is that you will continue to watch over this book too, that you will see the honesty and integrity you instilled in me blossom as I share my story with the goal of helping others. I heard you and I accept the assignment of this mountain so I can show others it can be moved.

Kathy Evans, you are a godsend. With great respect and patience, you helped me with the first round of edits to this book. You are very good at what you do! I'm grateful that our lives have so beautifully intersected again. Even though we are two provinces apart and mostly had to rely on video chats to work through the edits, sharing your unending support, insight and knowledge made the process enjoyable. I am not exaggerating when I say that I could not have brought this book to fruition without you. Thank you!

Jeanne Martinson, you too have been God sent. What are the chances that an unknown author in remote, southern Saskatchewan would find a skilled, successful publisher within a half hour of our home? Thank you for always working within my limitations and doing it with grace and patience. Thank you for the laughs and unending encouragement. Did you ever think you'd work with an author who couldn't read her own book? I will forever be grateful for all you've done to make this dream come true.

To my "beta readers" Trish Ireland, Liz Roberts, Alison Lewis, Leila Elder, Troy Rusu of the Saskatchewan Acquired Brain Injury support group and your team; thank you for taking time to read through the manuscript and provide honest and technical feedback. Your contribution is greatly appreciated.

Most importantly I thank God for always loving me, for never leaving me nor forsaking me, for allowing these experiences that shape the person He has always meant for me to be.

*"Brain injury, it's the last thing on your mind until it's the only thing"*

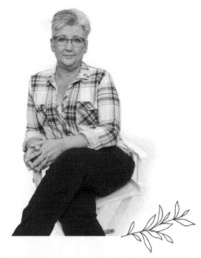

# Julianne Heagy
## Biography

Born in July, 1958 in Woodstock, Ontario, Julianne Peter was the third of five children born to two very loving, hardworking, entrepreneurial parents. Raised in the small community of Melbourne, Ontario, the author started her schooling in a one-room school and advanced to larger, multiroom schools in Glencoe, Ontario for her middle school years to grade 11.

Being an adventurous child, in her late teens, Julianne hopped on a train to Saskatchewan to help family friends with childcare needs. That began her love of western Canada and eventually she joined the family friends in Fife Lake, Saskatchewan and took her grade 12 at Rockglen

School in the neighbouring community. It was there she experienced her first brain injury from a car accident and, incidentally, met her husband, Blair Heagy.

In the following years, her work took her between Ontario and Saskatchewan. Career choices started as a server at Kentucky Fried Chicken, to the secretarial pool at Revenue Canada, then to a lengthy career in insurance, banking, and then as a medical records tech at various local hospitals. From 1997 to 2009, Julianne managed her own retail business that evolved from a gift shop into a day spa (all while continuing to work part time at local health facilities). In the years that followed, she continued to do remedial massage therapy from her home and work for the health district, finally taking on the position as a Member Relations Officer for a co-operative retail.

Having a natural curiosity, a sense of adventure and an affinity for learning, the author completed many courses and acquired several certifications: Office Education (Saskatchewan Technical Institute); Fellowship of the Life Management Institute with a specialty in Selection of Risk and Information Systems (computers, before they were in every office); Medical Record Technician (now Health Information Manager or HIM); Chartered Herbalist; Registered Massage Therapist; Low Intensity Laser Therapist; and a certificate in Commercial Credit Administration.

Always wanting to give back to her community, Julianne volunteered as a board member at her local Credit Union, stood as finance director for the Saskatchewan Women's Agricultural Network (SWAN), was the provincial president of the Massage Therapist Association of Saskatchewan (MTAS), was an active member of the Kinette organization for several years, and volunteering as needed in her community.

In 1988, she married her long-time best friend, Blair. In 1989, their son Jared was born and 18 months later in 1991, their daughter Justine completed their family.

In 2013, Blair was diagnosed with lung cancer which he successfully fought off. By 2015, the cancer returned, and he was deemed to have stage IV lung cancer with a rather poor prognosis. Julianne was torn between working multiple jobs to help supplement their reduced income and spending more time with her ill husband. Her ischemic stroke in 2019 took away many things she felt were important and that defined her—but also gave her the time with Blair she so desperately wanted. Blair continues to live day to day with his continuing stage IV prognosis and Julianne continues to live day to day with her acquired brain injury.

Made in the USA
Middletown, DE
25 February 2022